Study Guide for

Nursing Research in Canada: Methods, Critical Appraisal, and Utilization

Study Guide for

Nursing Research in Canada: Methods, Critical Appraisal, and Utilization

Fourth Canadian Edition

Geri LoBiondo-Wood, RN, PhD, FAAN
Professor and Coordinator, PhD in
Nursing Program University of Texas
Health Science Center at Houston
School of Nursing
Houston, Texas

Judith Haber, PhD, APRN, BC, FAAN
Ursula Springer Leadership Professor
in Nursing Associate Dean
for Graduate Programs
New York University
College of Nursing
New York, New York

Cherylyn Cameron, RN, PhD
Dean, School of Community Studies
and Creative Technologies
Bow Valley College
Calgary, Alberta

Mina D. Singh
Associate Director, Research
Associate Professor
School of Nursing
York University
Toronto, Ontario

Study Guide prepared by:

Carey A. Berry, MS, BSN, RN
Formerly, Clinical Nurse
Gastrointestinal Surgical Oncology
M.D. Anderson Cancer Center
The University of Texas
Denver, Colorado

Jennifer Yost, PhD, RN
Assistant Professor
School of Nursing, Faculty
of Health Sciences
McMaster University
Hamilton, Ontario

Joan Samuels-Dennis, RN, PhD
Adjunct Professor
School of Nursing
Trinity Western University
Langley, British Columbia
CEO, BECOMING Canada
jsdennis@becomingtrueself.com

ELSEVIER

ELSEVIER

Library and Archives Canada Cataloguing in Publication

Berry, Carey A., author
     Study guide for Nursing research in Canada : methods, critical appraisal, and utilization / Carey A. Berry (MS, BSN, RN, Formerly, Clinical Nurse, Gastrointestinal Surgical Oncology, M.D. Anderson Cancer Center, The University of Texas, Denver, Colorado), Jennifer Yost (PhD, RN, Assistant Professor, School of Nursing, Faculty of Health Sciences McMaster University, Hamilton, Ontario) ; Canadian editor: Joan Samuels-Dennis (RN, PhD, Assistant Professor, School of Nursing, Trinity Western University, Langley, British Columbia; Director, Trinity Centre Inc., Bolton, Ontario). — Fourth Canadian edition.

Includes bibliographical references and index.
Supplement to: Nursing research in Canada.
ISBN 978-1-77172-139-4 (softcover)

     1. Nursing—Research—Canada—Problems, exercises, etc. I. Yost, Jennifer, author II. Samuels-Dennis, Joan, 1973-, editor III. Title.

RT81.5.N8724 2017 Suppl.   610.73072'071   C2017-905009-5

Vice-President, Medical and Canadian Education: Madelene J. Hyde
Content Strategist: Roberta A. Spinosa-Millman
Senior Content Development Manager: Laurie Gower
Senior Content Development Specialist: Heather Bays
Project Manager: Radhika Sivalingam

Elsevier Canada
420 Main Street East, Suite 636,
Milton, ON Canada L9T 5G3
Phone: 1-416-644-7053

1 2 3 4 5 21 20 19 18 17
EBook ISBN: 978-1-77172-137-0

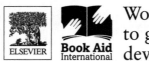

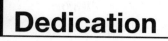

Dedication

I would like to thank Richard, Christopher, and Trinity for their continued support, without which this project would not have been possible. Thank you also to the students of Trinity Western University, Humber College, and York University, who offered valuable feedback on many of the activities outlined in this study guide.

Joan Samuels-Dennis

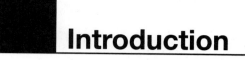

Introduction

In today's technologically advanced world, we are bombarded by information. The student's lament used to be, "I can't find any information on X." Now the cry is, "What do I do with all of the information on X?" The focus has shifted from how to find information to how to use information: What information is worth keeping? What should be discarded? What is useful to nursing practice? What is fluff? Where are the gaps?

Thinking about the links between information and practice is critical to the improvement of nursing care. As each of us in the field of nursing strengthens our understanding of the links between interventions and outcomes, we move nursing's collective practice closer to being truly evidence informed; we can "know" which intervention works best in which situation.

"Helping people get better" begins with critical thinking. The activities in this *Study Guide* are intended to strengthen your ability to think about information. The activities are designed to help you evaluate research reports and critically analyze research studies. As you practise the critiquing skills discussed in this *Study Guide*, you will be strengthening your ability to make practice-informed decisions that are grounded in nursing theory and research.

What an incredible time to be a nurse!

General Directions

1. We recommend that you read the textbook chapter first, and then complete the *Study Guide* activities for that chapter.
2. Complete each chapter, and the activities in each chapter, sequentially. The activities are designed to give you the opportunity to apply what you have learned from the textbook and actually use this knowledge to solve problems, thereby gaining the increased confidence that comes only from working through each chapter.
3. Follow the directions provided for each activity. Be certain that you have the resources needed to complete each activity before you begin that activity.
4. Complete the Post-Test after you have completed all of the chapter's activities. The answers for the Post-Tests can be obtained from your instructor. If you have answered 85% of the questions correctly, you can be confident that you have grasped the essential material presented in the chapter.
5. If you have any questions, confusion, or concerns, you can clarify these with your instructor.

Activity Answers

Answers in a study guide such as this are not "cut and dried" like the answers in a mathematics textbook. You will frequently be asked to make a "judgement call" about a particular problem. If your judgement differs from that of the authors, review the criteria you used to make your decision. Determine if you followed a logical progression of steps to reach your conclusion; if you think you did not, redo the activity. If the process you followed appears logical and your answer remains different from the authors' answer, remember that even experts disagree about many such judgement calls in nursing research. There will continue to be many "grey areas." Again, if you average 85% agreement with the authors, you are on the right track and should feel very confident about your level of expertise.

Carey A. Berry, MS, BSN, RN
Jennifer Yost, PhD, RN
Joan Samuels-Dennis, RN, PhD

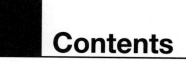

Contents

1 The Role of Research in Nursing

INTRODUCTION

One goal of this Study Guide chapter is to assist you in reviewing the material presented in Chapter 1 of *Nursing Research in Canada: Methods, Critical Appraisal, and Utilization.* A second and more fundamental goal is to provide you with an opportunity to begin practising the role of a critical consumer of research. Subsequent chapters in this study guide will strengthen your ability to evaluate research studies critically.

LEARNING OUTCOMES

On completion of this chapter, you will able to do the following:
- State the significance of research to the practice of nursing.
- Identify the role of the consumer of nursing research.
- Discuss the differences in trends in nursing research in Canada.
- Describe how research, education, and practice are related to each other.
- Evaluate the nurse's role in the research process as it relates to the nurse's level of education.
- Identify future trends in nursing research.
- Formulate the priorities for nursing research in the twenty-first century.

Activity 1

Match each term in Column B with the appropriate phrase in Column A. Each term will be used only once. (This may be a good time to review the textbook's glossary.)

Column A

1. _____ Systematic inquiry into possible relationships among particular phenomena

2. _____ One who reads critically and applies research findings in nursing practice

3. _____ Examination of the effects of nursing care on patient outcomes in a systematic process

4. _____ Critical evaluation of a research report's content, using a set of criteria to evaluate the scientific merit for application

5. _____ Implementation of a scientifically sound, research-based innovation into clinical practice

6. _____ Theoretical or pure research that generates tests and expands theories that explain phenomena

7. _____ Clinical practice based on the collection, interpretation, and integration of expert knowledge, research-derived evidence, and patient preferences

Column B

a. Critique

b. Consumer

c. Research

d. Clinical research

e. Basic research

f. Evidence-informed practice

g. Research utilization

Activity 2

Listed below are specific research activities. Indicate which academic degree is needed by nurses who have primary responsibility for each activity. Use the abbreviations provided by the key.

Key: A = baccalaureate degree C = doctoral degree
B = master's degree

1. _____ Designing and conducting research studies

2. _____ Identifying nursing problems that need investigation

3. _____ Assisting others in applying nursing's scientific knowledge

4. _____ Developing methods of scientific inquiry

5. _____ Assisting in data-collection activities

6. _____ Being a knowledgeable consumer of research

7. _____ Demonstrating an awareness of the value of nursing research

8. _____ Collaborating with experienced researchers in proposals, development, data analysis, and interpretation

9. _____ Promoting the integration of research into clinical practice

Activity 3

Complete the following crossword puzzle as you would any other crossword puzzle. Note that there will be no spaces between words in answers consisting of two or more words. Refer to the textbook as you complete the activity.

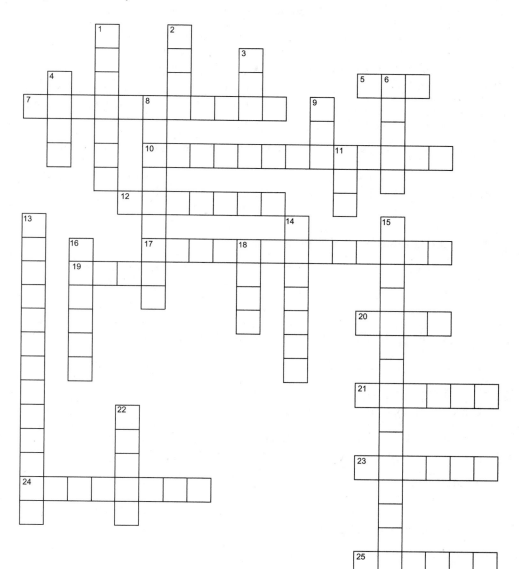

Across

5. Lobbying group (abbr.)
7. Possible result of a series of studies
10. Forerunner of *Canadian Journal of Nursing Research (CJNR)* (two words)
12. Limits nursing research
17. Nursing research priority (two words)
19. Nursing research association (abbr.)
20. Number of Canadian Health Services Research Foundation (CHSRF)/Canadian Institutes of Health Research (CIHR) nursing research chairs in 2000
21. Location of war from which Florence Nightingale collected data
23. Focus of nursing research
24. _____-informed practice
25. Research links and practice

Down

1. Name of a seminar on doctoral research
2. What research collects
3. Where the first master's program was offered (abbr.)
4. 1932 report that recommended better nursing education
6. Florence Nightingale's work
8. All nurses are research _____
9. Evidence-informed practice abbreviation
11. Published nursing research journal (abbr.)
13. 15 in Canada (two words)
14. Province with first PhD program
15. Journal published in 1952 (two words)
16. First centre for nursing research
18. Association representing nursing schools (abbr.)
22. Group that has historically been excluded from major research projects

Activity 4—Evidence-Informed Practice Activity

1. Reflect on what it was about nursing that prompted you to seek a baccalaureate degree.

_____

2. Reflect on one or two areas of nursing practice or groups of people that most interest you as you consider future job opportunities. Why do they interest you?

_____

3. Identify a research question that will help you address a problem in your identified areas of interest or that concerns the population with whom you wish to work. Important note: A research question should identify a problem of significance to nursing and the population likely to benefit from addressing the question, it should be open-ended, and it should allow for the use of a variety of methods to address the question. Consider reviewing Chapter 4 if this process piques your interest!

_____

4. Complete a simple Google search to see what types of nursing research have been done regarding your particular question. Did you find any interesting results?

_____

Activity 5—Web-Based Activity

Complete a Google Scholar search using the research question identified in Activity 4.

1. What types of nursing research have been done regarding your particular question?

2. Did you find any interesting results?

Activity 6

Answer the following questions in a way that is meaningful to you.

1. Why is knowing about nursing research important?

2. Keeping in mind your responses to the questions from Activity 5, how will nurse researchers produce depth in nursing knowledge concerning your identified areas or population of interest?

3. If you were asked to go on the *Dr. Oz* show to talk about nursing practice, what research information would you like to have to assist you in preparing for the interview?

POST-TEST

1. Listed below are descriptions of research activities carried out by nurses. In the space before each description, indicate (with the letters shown in the key) which degree a nurse should have for each activity.

   Key:
   A = baccalaureate degree
   B = master's degree
   C = doctoral degree

   a. _____ Providing expert consulting to a unit that is considering changing its practice on the care of decubitus ulcers on the basis of results from a series of studies

   b. _____ Measuring and recording the blood pressures of hypertensive patients during their monthly visits to the clinic, as part of a study on the effects of contingency contracting by a nurse researcher

   c. _____ Understanding and critically appraising research studies to determine whether a study is provocative or the findings have sufficient support to be considered for utilization

   d. _____ Designing and conducting research studies to expand nursing knowledge

2. Match each period listed in Column B with the appropriate event listed in Column A. (Not all answers in Column B are used.)

Column A

1. _____ First nursing doctoral program, begun at the University of Alberta

2. _____ Weir Report published

3. _____ Nightingale studied British mortality rates in the Crimean War

4. _____ Establishment of nursing research chairs

5. _____ *Nursing Research* first published

Column B

a. 1995 to 1999

b. Middle and late nineteenth century

c. 1991

d. 1932

e. 1992

f. 1952

g. 1900

h. 2000

Please check with your instructor for the answers to the Post-Test.

REFERENCE

Canadian Nurses Association. (2011). *The Next Decade: CNA's Vision for Nursing and Health.* Retrieved from http://www.cna-aiic.ca/cna/default_e.aspx

2 Theoretical Framework

INTRODUCTION

It is not uncommon for beginning students of research to find the theoretical part of a study to be their least favourite component. It tends to be heavily documented and is slow reading, but before long, you will find it a very valuable part of any study. The theoretical framework of a study provides you with the opportunity to see the research problem through the eyes of the researcher. As you read this section of a study, a window to the researcher's mind is opened; you get a glimpse of the way this particular researcher thinks about this particular problem. A critiquer's task is to consider respectfully the researcher's perspective, and then ask the following questions:

- How clearly do I understand the researcher's argument?
- Does the theoretical framework connect all of the pieces of the study?
- Can I see the relationship between the theoretical discussion and my clinical practice?

Most of the exercises in this chapter address the first question. Your ability to answer the second and third questions will improve as you complete the research course and as you build your clinical experience.

LEARNING OUTCOMES

On completion of this chapter, you will be able to do the following:
- Define key concepts in the philosophy of science.
- Identify and differentiate between theoretical/empirical, aesthetic, personal, sociopolitical, and ethical ways of knowing.
- Identify assumptions underlying the post-positivist, critical social, and interpretive/constructivist views of research.
- Compare inductive and deductive reasoning.
- Differentiate between conceptual and theoretical frameworks.
- Describe how a framework guides research.
- Differentiate between conceptual and operational definitions.
- Describe the relationships among theory, research, and practice.
- Discuss levels of abstraction related to frameworks guiding research.
- Describe the points of critical appraisal used to evaluate the appropriateness, cohesiveness, and consistency of a framework guiding research.

Activity 1

It is important to learn the vocabulary associated with research. Write definitions of the following terms, and be sure that you can differentiate between them.

a. Epistemology
b. Ontology

c. Concept
d. Theoretical framework
e. Paradigm
f. Constructivism
g. Post-positivism

Activity 2

In her important work, Carper (1978) described the four patterns of knowing pertinent to nursing as empirics, moral knowledge, personal knowing, and aesthetic knowing. Since then, several other nurse theorists, including Benner, Tanner, and Chesla (1992); Benner (2004); Chinn and Kramer (2015); and Zander (2007), have expanded on these ways of knowing. All of these authors suggest that no single way of knowing provides the entire truth, but instead offers simply a different perspective of the whole truth. These patterns of knowing can provide a foundation for a good understanding of the diversity and complexity of nursing. Nursing practice is guided by such knowledge. Rather than using instinct or intuition alone to determine knowledge, we use science in nursing because it is more reliable. Research is about asking good questions that generate knowledge. Questions asked by researchers are derived from a variety of philosophical positions.

a. What is the difference between theoretical and empirical knowledge? Provide an example of each.

_____

_____

_____

_____

Be sure you clearly understand the differences between quantitative and qualitative research, then write a clear definition of each of the following terms:

b. Quantitative research

_____

_____

_____

c. Qualitative research

_____

_____

_____

Activity 3

Review Table 2.1, Basic Beliefs of Research Paradigms, in your textbook, and compare the various premises of the constructivist paradigm with those of the post-positivist paradigm. Take some time to consider pain management as an important aspect of cancer care. Given what you already know about clinical care for this problem, suppose you wanted to learn more about the therapeutics of pain management for people with cancer who are largely cared for by family members. Suppose a case manager, hospice, or home health nurse wanted to facilitate excellence in pain management for a patient. Referring to Table 2.1, how might a researcher view the problem differently if he or she looked at it from a constructivist versus a positivist paradigm? Compare these two philosophical positions, and identify the differences between them. Try writing a research question for each paradigm related to this problem.

Activity 4

1. Jot down in your own words the defining characteristics of the following:

    a. Inductive thinking

    b. Deductive thinking

2. Play with these two kinds of thinking (inductive and deductive) before moving to the following clinical examples:

    a. Imagine you are hungry. You look around for something to eat. You find a decorative tin labelled "candy." You open the tin and see what looks like multicoloured oval beads. They sure do not look like any candies you have ever seen before, but you trust the person who would be putting things in this tin, so you decide to try them. Before long, you notice yourself looking for the mottled pink, orange, yellow, and black ones because these taste good. You leave the mottled yellow, white, and reddish-brown ones alone because you do not like them.

    Which term (*inductive* or *deductive*) best describes your activity?

    b. Sometime later, you feel those old hunger pangs returning. This time, the candy tin is empty. You want some more of those sweet multicoloured oval beads. You start thinking, "Those beads were in the candy tin. They were sweet. There is a candy store around the corner. I bet the candy store will have these sweet beads." You walk to the candy store and discover that your thinking was correct. The candy store does have those sweet beads, and they call them "jelly beans."

    Which term (*inductive* or *deductive*) best describes your thinking style in this situation?

3. Now think about the concept of "pain." More specifically, think about "headache pain." Picture several individuals (including yourself) experiencing a headache. List your observations.

Person 1	**Person 2**	**Person 3**	**Person 4**

Look at those observations. Do you see any similarities? Maybe a creased forehead? Rubbing temples with the fingertips? Rubbing the forehead? Rubbing the back of the neck? Grumpy? Preferring less light? Reaching for over-the-counter pain medication? Grimacing?

If you can, write a general statement about "signs of headache pain." If not, jot down your thoughts about why you are unable to write such a general statement.

Activity 5—Evidence-Informed Practice Activity

As explained in the text, concepts are the building blocks of a study. The greater the ease with which you can identify concepts, the easier it will become to analyze the theoretical framework of a given study. Once you can perform this analysis, you will be able to follow the line of logic from problem to conclusion.

1. Identify the concepts in each of the following excerpts from research:

   a. "The study investigated the efficacy of a medication administration Web course in increasing nursing students' self-evaluated competence on medication administration." (Mettiäinen, Luojus, Salminen, et al., 2014)

   b. "The study aims to describe undergraduate nurses'/midwives' perceptions of spirituality/spiritual care, their perceived competence in delivering spiritual care." (Ross, van Leeuwen, Baldacchino, et al., 2014)

   c. "This study prospectively monitored Swedish nursing students' burnout during the upper years of their nursing program and 1 year post-graduation." (Rudman & Gustavsson, 2012)

   d. "This study aims to test a large randomized controlled trial of an intervention directed to all disadvantaged youths in America to help them recognize difficult situations in which their automatic responses may be wrong." (Heller, Pollack, Ander, et al., 2013)

   e. "This study aims to examine the effectiveness of low-cost smoking interventions targeted to pregnant women and whether outcomes achieved with brief counseling from prenatal care providers and a self-help booklet could be improved by adding more resource-intensive cognitive-behavioral programs." (Ershoff, Quinn, Boyd, et al., 1999)

2. Now let's make things a bit more complex. Remember the definition of *concept*: It is an abstraction, a term that creates an image of an idea or some notion we want to share. Some concepts are more abstract than others. For example, *strain* is more abstract than *parental strain,* or *financial strain,* or *lumbar strain.* Frequently, the terms *concept* and *construct* are used interchangeably, but there is a subtle difference between them. Let's try to understand this a little better, using the *Concept Versus Construct* diagram below. In the diagram, *strain* is presented as a concept. Depending on your

professional background and life experiences, when you hear the word *strain,* a number of abstract ideas about what strain might mean pop into your head. *Strain* may represent difficulties that cause worry or emotional tension; injury to a muscle; or even a group of organisms of the same species that are slightly different genetically from one another. These ideas about what *strain* actually refers to are called *conceptual definitions.* Once we select a definition that truly corresponds with how we intend to view *strain,* we can identify the specific construct of interest. If we select the second definition—injury to a muscle—a number of other ideas pop into our head—for example, neck injury, lower-back injury, wrist, or shoulder injury. These concrete representations of strain are called *constructs.* A researcher interested in studying muscle injury as a form of strain could focus on one or all of the constructs listed in the *Concept Versus Construct* diagram.

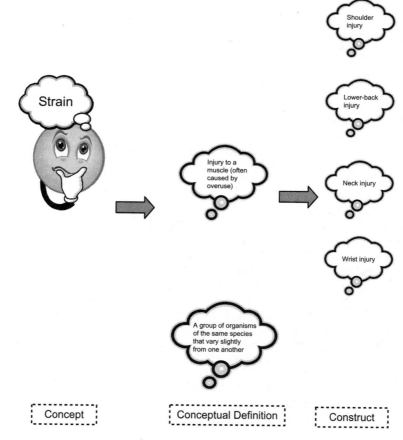

Concept Versus Construct

a. Which term—*health promotion* or *nursing diagnosis*—is a concept? Which is a construct?

b. Think about the concept and construct in the previous question. How are they alike?

c. How are they different?

3. Now it is your turn. Choose one concept from each of the five research examples in item 1 of this activity. Write a definition of the chosen concept using your own words.

a. _____

b. _____

c. _____

d. _____

e. _____

4. Compare your definition of the chosen concept with the definition of the same concept written by one of your peers. How close are your definitions? Think about the similarities and differences. Assume the two of you were going to work as co-investigators on a study that addressed the chosen concept.

a. What would you need to resolve?

b. Look one more time at those concepts. Do any of them more closely resemble a construct?

Activity 6

You have identified concepts, and you have written a definition of a concept. It is highly probable that the definition you wrote had more in common with a conceptual definition than with an operational definition. Operational definitions are a bit trickier. They outline the instrument or process that will be used to measure or observe a variable. They need to be so clear that you, the reader, have no questions about what the researcher meant by each concept/construct. Think about the concept of "verbal abuse." When you hear that term, what comes to mind? Manderino and Berkey (1997) defined *verbal abuse* as the score on "the Verbal Abuse Scale (VAS)." They went on to explain that the VAS is "a recently developed 65-item self-report questionnaire, clearly defining 11 different forms of verbal abuse, thus permitting a focused exploration of the frequency and perceived stressfulness of the various manifestations of abuse." The 11 categories of verbal abuse are ignoring, abusive anger, condescending, blocking/diverting, trivializing, abuse disguised as a joke, accusing/blaming, judging/criticizing, sexual harassment, discounting, and threatening.

Turn to the study by Laschinger (2014) in Appendix B and the study by Pauly, McCall, Browne, et al. (2015) in Appendix C of the textbook. Identify the conceptual and operational definitions in each of these studies. Do not expect every study to include both, and do not be surprised if some definitions are implicit rather than explicit.

Activity 7

Let's take a quick look at how theory, concepts, definitions, variables, and hypotheses fit together. There will be more details about variables and hypotheses in a later chapter, so the focus here is more on an understanding of how they are based in theory.

1. Match each term in Column B with the appropriate definition or example in Column A. Words in bold print in Column A indicate the element to be matched to a term. Items in Column B may be used more than once.

Column A

a. _____ "Fatigue symptoms were measured using the Modified Fatigue Symptoms Checklist (MFSC), a list of 30 symptoms of fatigue. Scores range from zero (no fatigue symptoms) to 30 symptoms (maximum fatigue)" (Milligan, Flenniken, & Pugh, 1996).

b. _____ ". . . **stress** and **empowerment** were used to guide this study" (Kendra, 1996).

c. _____ "Serenity is viewed as a learned, positive emotion of inner peace that can be sustained . . . that decreases perceived stress and improves physical and emotional health" (Roberts & Whall, 1996).

d. _____ Older (i.e., **more than 35 years of age**) first-time mothers (Reese & Harkless, 1996)

e. _____ Clinical decision making

f. _____ Quality of life

g. _____ "Acute confusion is a transient syndrome characterized primarily by abnormalities in attention and cognition, but disordered psychomotor behavior, sleep-wake disturbance, and autonomic nervous system disturbances are not uncommon" (Nellan, Champagne, Carlson, & Funk, 1996).

h. _____ "Are there **breathing pattern changes** from test to test or from the beginning to the end of the test?" (Hopp, Kim, Larson, & Sharp, 1996).

i. _____ "The combination of injury experience, knowledge, demographics, health beliefs, and social influence variables will predict home hazard accessibility" (Russell & Champion, 1996).

Column B

1. Variable

2. Hypothesis

3. Construct

4. Operational definition

5. Concept

6. Conceptual definition

2. This exercise gives you the opportunity to use all of the thinking you have done so far in tracing a variable from the introduction of a study through the theoretical rationale of that same study. Turn to Appendix B in the text and read the first part of the study conducted by Laschinger (2014). Read from the beginning of the study (including the title) to the section entitled "Methods." (Do not read the section on methods.)

   a. What type of reasoning is operating in this study?

   b. Were hypotheses developed for this study?

   c. Which of the following describes the theoretical rationale for this study?

   _____ A theoretical framework

   _____ A theory

   _____ A conceptual model

   _____ None of the above

POST-TEST

1. List three reasons that support the importance of the theoretical rationale of a study.

   a. _____

   b. _____

   c. _____

2. Read each of the statements below. Decide if each statement is true or false by marking it with a *T* if the statement is true and an *F* if the statement is false. Rewrite the false statements to make them true statements.

   a. _____ "Caregiving" is an example of a concept so clearly understood that there is no need for it to be operationally defined in a research study.

   b. _____ The following is an example of an operational definition: "The Beck Dressing Performance Scale (BDPS) (Beck, Heacock, Mercer, et al., 1997) was used to measure the major dependent variable, the level of caregiver assistance provided during dressing. The dressing function is broken down into 42 discrete component steps for males and 45 for females. A trained rater assigns each step of the dressing activity a score of 0 (independent) to 7 (complete dependence) based on the amount of assistance required to complete each step. Higher scores indicate greater dependence" (Beck et al., 1997).

   c. _____ The words printed in bold in the following phrase are the name of a construct: ". . . **define a professional practice model** (PPM) as a system that supports registered nurse control over the delivery of nursing care and the environment in which care is delivered" (Hoffart & Woods, 1997).

d. _____ The following is an example of a conceptual definition: "Although there is no standard definition of social support, there seems to be general acceptance of some basic typologies. House, Umberson, and Landis (1988) defined social support as positive dimensions of relationships that may promote health and buffer stress."

e. _____ The following is a sketch of a concept: ". . . verbal abuse was defined as verbal behaviors that are perceived as humiliating, degrading, and/or disrespectful. Because verbally abusive encounters potentially can be stressful, it seemed appropriate to address this issue within the framework of a model of stress . . . the major tenet of this model [sic: Lazarus' transactional model of stress coping] is that stress occurs in the face of perceived demands that tax or exceed the perceived coping resources of the person" (Manderino & Berkey, 1997).

3. Determine which of the following statements reflect the quantitative (qn) or qualitative (ql) research method.

a. _____ Statistical explanation, prediction, and control

b. _____ Neutral observer

c. _____ Multiple realities exist

d. _____ Objectivism valued

e. _____ Active participant

f. _____ Experimental

g. _____ Dialogic

h. _____ Time and place are important

i. _____ One reality exists

j. _____ Values add to understanding the phenomenon

Please check with your instructor for the answers to the Post-Test.

REFERENCES

Beck, C., Heacock, P., Mercer, S. O., et al. (1997). Improving dressing behavior in cognitively impaired nursing home residents. *Nursing Research, 46*(3), 126–132.

Benner, P. (2004). Using the Dreyfus model of skill acquisition to describe and interpret skill acquisition and clinical judgment in nursing practice and education. *Bulletin of Science, Technology & Society, 24*(3), 188.

Benner, P., Tanner, C., & Chesla, C. (1992). From beginner to expert: Gaining a differentiated clinical world in critical care nursing. *Advances in Nursing Science, 14*(3), 13.

Carper, B. (1978). Fundamental patterns of knowing in nursing. *Advanced Nursing Science, 1*(1), 13–23.

Chinn, P. L., & Kramer, M. K. (2015). *Knowledge development in nursing. Theory and process.* (9th ed.). St. Louis, MO: Elsevier.

Ershoff, D. H., Quinn, V. P., Boyd, N. R., et al. (1999). The Kaiser Permanente Prenatal Smoking-Cessation Trial: When more isn't better, what is enough? *American Journal of Preventive Medicine, 17*(3), 161–168.

Heller, S., Pollack, H. A., Ander, R., et al. (2013). Preventing youth violence and dropout: A randomized field experiment (No. w19014). National Bureau of Economic Research.

Hoffart, N., & Woods, C. Q. (1997). Elements of a nursing professional practice model. *Journal of Professional Nursing, 12*(6), 354–364.

Hopp, L. J., Kim, M. J., Larson, J. L., et al. (1996). Incremental threshold loading in patients with chronic obstructive pulmonary disease. *Nursing Research, 45*(4), 196–202.

House, J. S., Umberson, D., & Landis, K. R. (1988). Structures and processes of social support. *Annual Review of Sociology, 14*, 293–318.

Kendra, M. A. (1996). Perception of risk by home health care administrators and field workers. *Public Health Nursing, 13*(6), 386–393.

Laschinger, H. K. S. (2014). Impact of workplace mistreatment on patient safety risk and nurse-assessed patient outcomes. Journal of Nursing Administration, 44(5), 284–290.

Manderino, M. A., & Berkey, N. (1997). Verbal abuse of staff nurses by physicians. *Journal of Professional Nursing, 13*(1), 48–55.

Mettiäinen, S., Luojus, K., Salminen, S., et al. (2014). Web course on medication administration strengthens nursing students' competence prior to graduation. *Nurse Education in Practice, 14*(4), 368–373.

Milligan, R. A., Flenniken, P. M., & Pugh, L. C. (1996). Positioning intervention to minimize fatigue in breastfeeding women. *Applied Nursing Research, 9*(2), 67–70.

Nellan, V. J., Champagne, M. T., Carlson, J. R., et al. (1996). The NEECHAM confusion scale: Construction, validation, and clinical testing. *Nursing Research, 45*(6), 324–330.

Pauly, B., McCall, J., Browne, A. J., et al. (2015). Toward cultural safety: Nurse and patient perceptions of illicit substance use in a hospitalized setting. *Advances in Nursing Science, 38*(2), 121–135.

Reese, S. M., & Harkless, G. (1996). Clinical methods: Divergent themes in maternal experience in women older than 35 years of age. *Applied Nursing Research, 9*(3), 148–153.

Roberts, K. T., & Whall, A. (1996). Serenity as a goal for nursing practice. *Image: Journal of Nursing Scholarship, 28*(4), 359–364.

Ross, L., van Leeuwen, R., Baldacchino, D., et al. (2014). Student nurses perceptions of spirituality and competence in delivering spiritual care: A European pilot study. *Nurse Education Today, 34*(5), 697–702.

Rudman, A., & Gustavsson, J. P. (2012). Burnout during nursing education predicts lower occupational preparedness and future clinical performance: A longitudinal study. *International Journal of Nursing Studies, 49*(8), 988–1001.

Russell, K. M., & Champion, V. L. (1996). Health beliefs and social influence in home safety practices of mothers with preschool children. *Image: Journal of Nursing Scholarship, 28*(1), 59–64.

Zander, P. E. (2007). Ways of knowing in nursing: The historical evolution of a concept. *Journal of Theory Construction and Testing, 11*(1), 7–11.

3 Critical Reading Strategies: Overview of the Research Process

INTRODUCTION

Tools are needed for whatever task one sets out to do. Sometimes, the tools are relatively simple and concrete (e.g., a pencil). At other times, the tools are abstract and more difficult to describe. The tools you need to in order critically consider research fit into the category of abstract tools and are tools of the mind (e.g., tools for critical thinking and reading). The following activities are designed to help you recognize and use these tools.

LEARNING OUTCOMES

On completion of this chapter, you will be able to do the following:
- Identify the steps that researchers use to conduct quantitative and qualitative research.
- Identify the importance of critical thinking and critical reading for the reading of research articles.
- Identify the steps associated with critical reading.
- Use the steps of critical reading to review research articles.
- Use identified strategies to critically read research articles.
- Use identified critical thinking and critical reading strategies to synthesize critiqued articles.
- Identify the format and style of research articles.

Activity 1

Complete the statements in items 1 and 2 below with one of the two words presented in parentheses. Complete the statements in items 3, 4, and 5 with the appropriate word or phrase from the text.

1. Critical thinking is a(n) _____ (rational; irrational) process.

2. Paul and Elder (2008) state that critical thinking is a(n) _____ (active; passive), intellectually engaging process in which the reader participates in an _____ (inner; outer) dialogue with the writer.

3. To read critically, readers must enter the point of view of someone other than themselves; specifically, they must enter _____.

4. Nursing students are first introduced to critical thinking skills through use of the _____ processes of assessment, diagnosis, planning, intervention, and evaluation.

5. The minimum number of readings of a research article as recommended in the text is _____.

Activity 2

Match each phrase in Column A with the appropriate term from Column B. Terms from Column B will be used more than once.

Column A

Column B

a. Critical thinking

b. Critical reading

1. _____ Getting a general sense of the material

2. _____ Clarifying unfamiliar terms within the text

3. _____ Using constructive skepticism

4. _____ Questioning assumptions

5. _____ Examining ideas rationally

6. _____ Thinking about your own thinking

Activity 3

1. The process of critical reading has four levels (or stages) of understanding. The levels are listed below in a scrambled order. Rearrange them in the correct order and write them in the blanks below.

   Scrambled order:
   Synthesis understanding
   Preliminary understanding
   Comprehensive understanding
   Analysis understanding

   Appropriate order:

   a. _____

   b. _____

   c. _____

   d. _____

2. Synthesis understanding, or "putting it all together," is one of the final steps in critical reading. It can be broken down into a series of activities that work best if completed in order. The steps are listed below in a scrambled order. Rearrange them in the appropriate order and write them in the blanks below.

   Scrambled order:
   Staple the summary to the top of the copied article.
   Summarize the study in your own words.
   Complete one handwritten index/cue card per study.
   Review your notes on the copy.
   Read the article for the fourth time.

Appropriate order:

a. _____

b. _____

c. _____

d. _____

e. _____

Activity 4

Determine whether the articles in Appendix C (Pauly, McCall, Browne, et al., 2015) and Appendix D (Héon, Goulet, Garofalo, et al., 2016) of the text are quantitative or qualitative studies. Use the following points to determine if the study you are reading is of a quantitative design. First, check off "Yes" or "No" after each item and then summarize your thoughts in a paragraph.

Criteria	Appendix C	Appendix D
1. Hypotheses are stated or implied in the article.	☐ Yes ☐ No	☐ Yes ☐ No
2. The terms *control group* and *treatment group* appear.	☐ Yes ☐ No	☐ Yes ☐ No
3. One of these terms—*checklist, survey, correlational*, or *ex post facto*—is used. (*Note:* Read the glossary definitions for help in answering this question.)	☐ Yes ☐ No	☐ Yes ☐ No
4. The terms *random* and *convenience* are mentioned in relation to the sample.	☐ Yes ☐ No	☐ Yes ☐ No
5. Variables are measured by instruments or tools.	☐ Yes ☐ No	☐ Yes ☐ No
6. The reliability and validity of instruments are discussed.	☐ Yes ☐ No	☐ Yes ☐ No
7. Statistical analyses are used.	☐ Yes ☐ No	☐ Yes ☐ No

Summary for Appendix C:

_____

_____

_____

_____

_____

Summary for Appendix D:

_____

_____

_____

_____

_____

Activity 5—Web-Based Activity

Go to the website at http://www.criticalthinking.org (Foundation for Critical Thinking, 2011). Under the "Library" tab, click on "About Critical Thinking," and read the following articles:
- Defining Critical Thinking
- A Brief History of the Idea of Critical Thinking
- Sumner's Definition of Critical Thinking
  a. Which one of the three articles did you like best?
  b. What did you learn from the article that you liked best?
  c. List your strengths in critical thinking. Are you open to new experiences and new ways of looking at "problems"? Think about this, and assess your strengths.
  d. In what areas of critical thinking do you need to improve?

Activity 6—Evidence-Informed Practice Activity

Read the statements in Column A (excerpts from published journal articles). Match the correct response from Column B (steps in the research process) to the statement in Column A. Note that not all responses in Column B are used.

Column A

1. _____ "As women faced the possibility of pregnancy complication, painful daily injections, and perceived lack of a professional support, they exemplified remarkable resourcefulness in taking control and taking steps to meet their needs" (Martens & Emed, 2007, p. 59).

2. _____ "In order to explore the technology readiness of nursing and medical study, the 2006 cohorts of medical and nursing students at Memorial University of Newfoundland (MUN) were studied, using a cross-sectional survey approach" (Caison, Bulma, Pai, et al., 2008, p. 285).

3. _____ "Further research is planned with larger sample size to confirm these results" (Caison et al., 2008, pp. 209–291).

4. _____ "Thrombophilia is a serious hypercoagulability disorder that contributes to maternal mortality and has been associated with significant pregnancy complication including intrauterine growth restriction, preeclampsia, and recurrent fetal loss" (Martens & Emed, 2007, p. 55).

5. _____ "Thematic analysis was used throughout the process of interviewing, transcribing and reviewing the data. Transcripts and field notes were examined line by line and key statements regarding participants' experiences highlighted and coded" (Martens & Emed, 2007, p. 57).

Column B

1. Identify research purpose and question

2. Review and critique existing literature

3. Identify guiding theoretical framework

4. Determine study design

5. Select sample

6. Measure concepts of interest

7. Data analysis

8. Report finding

POST-TEST

1. When analyzing research articles, it is important to remember that the researcher may _____ (omit, vary) the steps but that the steps must still be systematically addressed.

2. To critically read a research study, you must have skilled reading, writing, and reasoning abilities. Read the following excerpt from an abstract, then identify concepts, clarify any unfamiliar concepts or terms, and question any assumptions or rationales presented.

   This article describes risky drug and sexual behavior and mental health characteristics in a sample of 240 homeless or drug-recovering women and their most immediate sources of social support. . . . Fifty-one percent of the women and 31% of their support sources had Center for Epidemiological Studies Depression Scale (CES-D) scores of 27 or greater, suggesting a high level of depressive disorders in both samples. Similarly, 76% of the women and 59% of their support sources had psychological well-being scores below a standard clinical cut-off point. These data suggest that homeless and impoverished women turn to individuals who are themselves at high risk for emotional distress and risky behaviours as their main sources of support (Nyamathi, Flaskerud, & Leake, 1997).

a. Identify concepts.

b. List any unfamiliar concepts or terms that you would need to clarify.

c. List the questions you would ask regarding assumptions or rationales.

3. Quantitative and qualitative articles in journals vary a great deal in format and style. The following statements will focus your attention on these differences and help you distinguish between the two major types of research. Complete each statement by inserting the correct terms from the list below. Not every term will be used.

used

conducted

generate hypotheses

test a hypothesis

statistical tests

analyze themes or concepts

a. The primary difference between the two types of study is that the qualitative study does not

_____ but may _____.

b. An additional major difference is in the way literature reviews are _____

and _____ in the study.

Please check with your instructor for the answers to the Post-Test.

REFERENCES

Caison, A. L., Bulman, D., Pai, S., et al. (2008). Exploring the technology readiness of nursing and medical students at a Canadian university. *Journal of Interprofessional Care, 22*(3), 283–294.

Foundation for Critical Thinking. (2011). *About critical thinking.* Retrieved from http://www.critical-thinking.org

Héon, M., Goulet, C., Garofalo, C., Nuyt, A.M. & Levy, E. (2016). An intervention to promote breast milk production in mothers of preterm infants. *Western Journal Of Nursing Research, 38*(5), 529–552.

Martens, T. Z., & Emed, J. D. (2007). The experiences and challenges of pregnant women coping with thrombophilia. *Journal of Obstetric, Gynecologic, & Neonatal Nursing, 36*(1), 55–62.

Nyamathi, A., Flaskerud, J., & Leake, B. (1997). HIV-risk behaviors and mental health characteristics among homeless or drug-recovering women and their closest sources of social support. *Nursing Research, 46*(3), 133–137.

Paul, R., & Elder, L. (2008). *The miniature guide to critical thinking concepts and tools*. Dillon Beach, CA: Foundation for Critical Thinking Press.

Pauly, B., McCall, J., Browne, A.J., Parker, J., & Mollison, A. (2015). Toward cultural safety: Nurse and patient perceptions of illicit substance use in a hospitalized setting. *Advances in Nursing Science, 38*(2),121–135.

4 Developing Research Questions, Hypotheses, and Clinical Questions

INTRODUCTION

This chapter focuses on the research question and hypothesis. When written correctly, a research question can be very helpful to you as a consumer of nursing research because it describes the essence of the research study concisely (usually in one or two sentences). For the nurse who considers using the results of a given study in practice, the two primary concerns are to locate the research question and to critique it. The hypothesis or the research question provides the most succinct link between the underlying theoretical base and the research design. Thus, its analysis is pivotal to the analysis of the entire research study.

LEARNING OUTCOMES

On completion of this chapter, you will be able to do the following:
- Discuss the purpose of developing a research question.
- Describe how the research question and hypothesis are related to the other components of the research process.
- Describe the process of identifying and refining a research question.
- Identify the criteria for determining the significance of a research question.
- Discuss the appropriate use of the purpose, aim, or objective of a research study.
- Discuss how the purpose, research question, and hypothesis suggest which level of evidence is to be obtained from the findings of a research study.
- Identify the characteristics of research questions and hypotheses.
- Describe the advantages and disadvantages of directional and nondirectional hypotheses.
- Compare the use of statistical hypotheses with that of research hypotheses.
- Discuss the appropriate use of research questions versus hypotheses in a research study.
- Discuss the differences between a research question and a clinical question in relation to evidence-informed practice.
- Identify the criteria used for critiquing a research question and a hypothesis.
- Apply the critiquing criteria to the evaluation of a research question and a hypothesis in a research report.

Activity 1

Match each term in Column B to the appropriate statement in Column A. Not all terms from Column B will be used.

Column A

1. _____ An interrogative sentence or declarative statement about the relationship between two or more variables.

2. _____ The variable that is the consequence or the presumed effect that varies with a change in the second variable.

3. _____ The variable that is manipulated in experimental research.

4. _____ The variable that is presumed to exist and is observed.

5. _____ A property of the problem that indicates it is measurable by either qualitative or quantitative methods.

6. _____ The properties that the researcher studies.

Column B

a. Testability

b. Independent variable

c. Variables

d. Dependent variable

e. Research question

f. Hypothesis

Activity 2

A good quantitative research question exhibits the following four characteristics:

a. It clearly and unambiguously identifies the variables under consideration.
b. It clearly expresses the variables and the expected relationship of the variables.
c. It specifies the nature of the population being studied.
d. It implies the possibility of empirical testing.

Examine the excerpts below to determine if each of the above criteria is present. Following each excerpt is a list representing the four criteria (a to d) listed above. Mark "Yes" or "No" to indicate whether each criterion is met.

  Study A: "The objective of this study was to determine the cost and effectiveness of a transitional discharge model (TDM) of care with clients who have a chronic mental illness" (Forchuk, Martin, Chan, et al., 2005).

  Study B: "The purpose of this study was to extend our understanding of employment status as a social determinant of psychological distress among single mothers" (Samuels-Dennis, 2006).

  Study C: "The project examines the impact of interprofessional education and collaboration interventions on interprofessional relationships, health care processes (including evidence-based practice), and patient outcomes" (Zwarenstein & Reeves, 2006).

	Criterion a	Criterion b	Criterion c	Criterion d
Forchuk et al., 2005	☐ Yes ☐ No	☐ Yes ☐ No	☐ Yes ☐ No	☐ Yes ☐ No
Samuels-Dennis, 2006	☐ Yes ☐ No	☐ Yes ☐ No	☐ Yes ☐ No	☐ Yes ☐ No
Zwarenstein & Reeves, 2006	☐ Yes ☐ No	☐ Yes ☐ No	☐ Yes ☐ No	☐ Yes ☐ No

Activity 3

Distinguishing between independent and dependent variables is a crucial preliminary step in determining whether a research hypothesis is a succinct statement of the relationship between two variables. Identify the variables in the following examples. Decide which is the independent (presumed cause) variable and which is the dependent (presumed effect) variable.

1. The use of cathode ray terminals (CRTs) increases the incidence of birth defects.

    a. Independent variable:

    b. Dependent variable:

2. Individuals with birth defects have a higher incidence of independence–dependence conflicts than individuals without birth defects.

    a. Independent variable:

    b. Dependent variable:

3. What is the relationship between daily moderate consumption of white wine and serum cholesterol levels?

    a. Independent variable:

    b. Dependent variable:

4. Problem-oriented recording leads to more effective patient care than narrative recording.

    a. Independent variable:

    b. Dependent variable:

5. Nurses and physicians differ in the way they view the extended-role concept for nurses.

   a. Independent variable:

   b. Dependent variable:

Activity 4

Now take each hypothesis or research question and label it in the blank space with the appropriate abbreviation from the following key. More than one abbreviation may be used to describe each item.

Key: RQ = research question
DH = directional hypothesis
NDH = nondirectional hypothesis
Hr = research hypothesis
Ho = statistical hypothesis

1. _____ The use of cathode ray terminals (CRTs) increases the incidence of birth defects.

2. _____ Individuals with birth defects have a higher incidence of independence–dependence conflicts than individuals without birth defects.

3. _____ What is the relationship between daily moderate consumption of white wine and serum cholesterol levels?

4. _____ Problem-oriented recording leads to more effective patient care than narrative recording.

5. _____ Nurses and physicians differ in the way they view the extended-role concept for nurses.

Activity 5

The next step is to practise writing hypotheses of different types. Return to the first three of the five hypotheses, questions, or problems you labelled in Activity 4. Each was labelled as a specific type of hypothesis or research question. Rewrite each of these first three to meet the conditions of the remaining four types of questions or hypotheses. The first problem is partially completed to provide an example.

1. The use of CRTs increases the incidence of birth defects.

   DH: The use of CRTs increases the incidence of birth defects.

   NDH: The use of CRTs influences the incidence of birth defects.

   Hr: The use of CRTs increases the incidence of birth defects.

   RQ:

   Ho:

2. Individuals with birth defects have a higher incidence of independence–dependence conflicts than individuals without birth defects.

   DH:

   NDH:

   Hr:

   RQ:

   Ho:

3. What is the relationship between daily moderate consumption of white wine and serum cholesterol levels?

   DH:

   NDH:

   Hr:

   RQ:

   Ho:

Activity 6

Critique the following hypotheses. (Two hypotheses were tested in this study.)

1. **Hypothesis I:** There will be significant improvement in the independent activities of daily living of cognitively impaired children (ages 5–10 years) following the implementation of the program to promote independence.

   a. Is the hypothesis clearly stated in a declarative form?

   ☐ Yes   ☐ No

   b. Are the independent and dependent variables identified in the statement of the hypothesis?

   ☐ Yes   ☐ No

   c. Are the variables measurable or potentially measurable?

   ☐ Yes   ☐ No

d. Is the hypothesis stated in such a way that it is testable?

☐ Yes   ☐ No

e. Is the hypothesis stated objectively without value-laden words?

☐ Yes   ☐ No

f. Is the direction of the relationship in the hypothesis clearly stated?

☐ Yes   ☐ No

2. **Hypothesis II:** There will be no difference in the time required by parents to complete activities of daily living with cognitively impaired children before and after implementing the program to promote independence.

a. Is the hypothesis clearly stated in a declarative form?

☐ Yes   ☐ No

b. Are the independent and dependent variables identified in the statement of the hypothesis?

☐ Yes   ☐ No

c. Are the variables measurable or potentially measurable?

☐ Yes   ☐ No

d. Is the hypothesis stated in such a way that it is testable?

☐ Yes   ☐ No

e. Is the hypothesis stated objectively without value-laden words?

☐ Yes   ☐ No

f. Is the direction of the relationship in the hypothesis clearly stated?

☐ Yes   ☐ No

g. Is each of the hypotheses specific to one relationship so that each hypothesis can be either supported or not supported?

☐ Yes   ☐ No

Activity 7—Evidence-Informed Practice Activity

You are designing a study for your research course. You would like to study the introduction of patient care technicians as team members to replace the primary care nursing model and its effect on patient outcomes in a cardiac unit. When deciding to conduct research, it is important to determine whether the topic is significant enough to study. Would the proposed outcomes study meet the criteria for being considered significant? Answer "yes" or "no," and then give the rationale underlying your choice.

Activity 8

As research has become an essential component to the provision of effective and safe health care, nurses are encouraged to be more familiar with research design, and make evidence-informed decisions in their clinical practice. The development of a well-defined research question, including a supportive hypothesis, is a key step in generating clinically relevant results to be used in evidence-informed practice. Review the online resource available at https://www.socialresearchmethods.net/kb/index.php to increase your understanding of important considerations in the development of a research question and hypothesis for research. Click on "Foundations" on the top left of the web page, then go to "Language of Research"; you will find some useful hyperlinks relevant to the major issues in research. Read through the information related to Types of Questions and Hypotheses, and answer the following question:

Explain the method to determine whether a sentence is a research question or a hypothesis.

POST-TEST

1. Choose the terms from the key provided below that best describe items a through h. Write the appropriate abbreviation(s) in the space provided. More than one abbreviation may be used to describe each item.

Key: RQ = research question
DH = directional hypothesis
NDH = nondirectional hypothesis
Hr = research hypothesis
Ho = statistical hypothesis

a. _____ There will be no change in self-rated body image among women in the three patient groups.

b. _____ What is the relationship between organizational climate dimensions and job satisfaction of nurses in neonatal intensive care units?

c. _____ The higher the perceived parental support, the lower is girls' general fearfulness.

d. _____ There will be a significant difference in pre-test and post-test results measuring the cognitive development level between undergraduate nursing students who have completed a research course and those who have not.

e. _____ The post-test mean of selected psychological variables for the experimental group will be lower than that of the control group.

f. _____ There will be no association found between the level of social support and self-care health practices.

g. _____ The educational preparation of a nurse (e.g., associate, diploma, BScN) will affect his or her ability to conduct thorough patient interviews.

h. _____ What is the level of postoperative infection following the use of clean tracheotomy care?

2. Fill in the blanks in the sentences below with the appropriate word or words from the list provided. Not every word in the list will be used.

research hypotheses	declarative statement
null hypotheses	nondirectional research hypothesis
predicts	directional research hypothesis
validity	population
testing	

a. The hypothesis is a vehicle for _____ the _____ of the assumptions of the theoretical framework of a research study.

b. A hypothesis transposes the question posed by the research problem into a _____ that _____ the relationship between two or more variables.

c. _____ are more common than _____ in studies that use deductive reasoning.

d. The _____ is a well-defined set that has certain properties that are often either specified or implied in the research question.

Please check with your instructor for the answers to the Post-Test.

REFERENCES

Forchuk, C., Martin, M. L., Chan, Y. L., & Jensen, E. (2005). Therapeutic relationships: From psychiatric hospital to community. *Journal of Psychiatric and Mental Health Nursing, 12,* 556–564.

Samuels-Dennis, J. (2006). Relationship among employment status, stressful life events, and depression in single mothers. *Canadian Journal of Nursing Research, 38*(1), 58–80.

Zwarenstein, M., & Reeves, S. (2006). Knowledge translation and interprofessional collaboration: Where the rubber of evidence-based care hits the road of teamwork. *Journal of Continuing Education in the Health Professions, 26*(1), 46–54.

5 Finding and Appraising the Literature

INTRODUCTION

The terms *review of the literature* and *literature review* most commonly refer to that section of a research study report where the researcher describes the link between knowledge found previously and the current study. Other research-related uses of a review of the literature are the following:
1. Developing an overall impression of the research and clinical work that have been done in a given area
2. Helping to clarify the research problem
3. Polishing research design ideas
4. Finding possible strategies for data collection and analysis

This chapter will help you learn more about each of these uses of literature review and provide you with the basic information you need in order to decide whether the researcher has thoroughly reviewed the relevant literature and used the review to its fullest potential.

LEARNING OUTCOMES

On completion of this chapter, you will be able to do the following:
- Discuss the relationship of the literature review to nursing theory, research, education, and practice.
- Discuss the purposes of the literature review for research projects and for evidence-informed projects.
- Differentiate between primary and secondary sources.
- Compare the advantages and disadvantages of the most commonly used online databases and print database sources for conducting a literature review.
- Identify the characteristics of an effective electronic search of the literature.
- Critically read, appraise, and synthesize primary and secondary sources used for the development of a literature review.
- Apply critiquing criteria to the evaluation of literature reviews in selected research studies.

Activity 1

The review of the literature is essential to the growth of nursing *theory*, *research*, *education*, and *practice*. Complete the sentences below with the appropriate italicized terms from the previous sentence to show what a critical review of the literature does.

1. Reveals appropriate _____ questions for the discipline

2. Provides the latest knowledge for _____.

3. Uncovers _____ findings that can lead to changes in clinical _____.

4. Uncovers new knowledge that can lead to the refinement of _____.

Activity 2

Listed below are examples of uses of the literature for research consumers in educational and practice settings. Match each type of research consumer in Column B with the activities listed in Column A. (Terms in Column B may be used more than once.)

Column A: Activities

1. _____ Implementing research-based nursing interventions

2. _____ Developing scholarly academic papers

3. _____ Developing practice guidelines

4. _____ Developing research proposals for master's theses

5. _____ Evaluating hospital continuous quality improvement programs

6. _____ Revising curricula

Column B: Research Consumer Types

a. Undergraduate students

b. Faculty members

c. Nurses in clinical settings

d. Graduate students

e. Governmental agencies

f. Professional nursing organizations

Activity 3

Researchers who are also clinicians are interested in solving clinical problems, whether the solutions are for immediate or future use. When faced with a problem in clinical practice, a clinician's first thought is often, "What have others learned about this problem?" To seek an answer to that question, the clinician usually goes first to the nursing literature. List five nursing journals that publish reports or research studies that you as a clinician might study to find out more about a problem.

1. _____

2. _____

3. _____

4. _____

5. _____

Activity 4

Usually, a review of the literature is easy to find in a journal article. In an abridged version of a research report, it is clearly labelled. Most frequently, one of the early sections of the report is labelled "Review of Literature" or "Relevant Literature" or some other comparable title. It may also be separated into a literature review section and another section (often entitled "Conceptual Framework") that presents the theoretical or conceptual framework on which the study is based. (Note: The length of the literature review section in a journal article varies. A range of two to several paragraphs is most common.)

1. Examine the article by Pauly, McCall, Browne, et al. (2015) in Appendix C and the article by Héon, Goulet, Garofalo, et al. (2016) in Appendix D of the textbook. What title is given to the literature review section of each of these articles (listed below)?

2. Assess the quality of literature review using the questions provided in the table below. For each article check "yes" or "no" in response to the questions being asked and provide a summary statement concerning the strengths and limitations of the literature review section of each article found in Appendices C and D.

Critical Appraisal of Literature Review				
Question	**Pauly et al.**		**Héon et al.**	
1. Does the author clearly identify the relevant concepts and/or variables being looked at in the study?	☐ Yes	☐ No	☐ Yes	☐ No
2. Is enough information given for you to assess if the search strategy included an appropriate and adequate number of research and theoretical sources?	☐ Yes	☐ No	☐ Yes	☐ No
3. Does an appropriate theoretical or conceptual framework guide the development of the research study?	☐ Yes	☐ No	☐ Yes	☐ No
4. Are mainly primary sources used?	☐ Yes	☐ No	☐ Yes	☐ No
5. Does the literature review uncover gaps or inconsistencies in knowledge?	☐ Yes	☐ No	☐ Yes	☐ No
6. Does the literature review build on the findings of earlier studies?	☐ Yes	☐ No	☐ Yes	☐ No
7. Does the critique of each reviewed study mention strengths, weaknesses, or limitations of the design; conflicts; and gaps in information related to the area of interest?	☐ Yes	☐ No	☐ Yes	☐ No
8. Is the literature review presented in an organized format that flows logically?	☐ Yes	☐ No	☐ Yes	☐ No
9. Does the literature review follow the proposed purpose of the research study or evidence-informed practice project?	☐ Yes	☐ No	☐ Yes	☐ No
10. Does the literature review generate research questions or hypotheses or answer a clinical question?	☐ Yes	☐ No	☐ Yes	☐ No

a. Summary of strengths and limitations for Pauly et al. (2015):

_____

_____

_____

_____

b. Summary of strengths and limitations for Héon et al. (2016):

_____

_____

_____

_____

3. Return to the article by Pauly et al. (2015). Determine how recent the articles listed in the reference section are. There should be some from the last 3 to 5 years, and they should show the development of the research over time. The whole article should read like a good detective story. At first, there may be qualitative studies that attempt to identify which variables are important to this problem or paradigm. At some point, you should also see researchers progressively analyze each of the variables, gradually narrowing and defining the scope of the problem, while others continue to look at the problem qualitatively. Do you see this in the literature and reference sections of this article?

Critique the currency of the references. Write the "story" you see in the reference section and in the review of the literature.

Activity 5

It is sometimes difficult to understand the distinction between primary and secondary sources of information. Here is an example of a helpful comparison: if you are considering giving a client an injection for pain, whose report would you feel most comfortable evaluating—the report of a family member or nurse's aide (i.e., a secondary source), or the report by the client (i.e., a primary source)? As a consumer of nursing research, you also need to evaluate the credibility of research designs and reports with respect to whether they have been generated from primary or secondary sources (i.e., whether the information you are reading is a first-hand report or someone else's interpretation of the material).

1. The following words or phrases describe either primary or secondary sources. Put a P next to those describing primary sources and an S next to those describing secondary sources.

a. _____ Summaries of research studies

b. _____ First-hand accounts

c. _____ Biographies

    d. _____ Textbooks

    e. _____ Client records

    f. _____ Reports written by the researcher

    g. _____ Dissertations or master's theses

2. The best source for primary research studies is the World Wide Web.

    □ True   □ False

3. You have access at home to the Cumulative Index to Nursing and Allied Health Literature (CINAHL) database and can now do your literature search without any additional cost.

    □ True   □ False

4. Information about CINAHL products and links to other nursing sources can be accessed at http://www.ebscohost.com/cinahl/.

    □ True   □ False

5. Which of the following is the best database for a search of nursing literature?

    a. MEDLINE

    b. CINAHL

    Why is it better than the other for searching nursing literature?

6. Print databases, such as the CINAHL print index, must be used for literature searches of material published before 1982.

    □ True   □ False

7. There is usually an extra charge for accessing the full text of an article from databases such as CINAHL.

    □ True   □ False

Activity 6

Below is a selected list of references from the article by Pauly et al. (2015) (Appendix C in the textbook). Next to each, indicate whether the reference is a primary *(P)* or secondary *(S)* source. Sometimes it is helpful to return to the text of the article and read the discussion of the reference; this may quickly tell you the type of article that is referenced.

1. _____ Galea, S., & Vlahov, D. (2002). Social determinants and the health of drug users: Socioeconomic status, homelessness and incarceration. *Public Health Reports, 117*(Suppl. 1), S135–S145.

2. _____ Browne, A. J., Smye, V. L., Rodney, P., et al. (2011). Access to primary care from the perspective of Aboriginal patients at an urban emergency department. *Qualitative Health Research, 21*(3), 333–348.

3. _____ Link, B., & Phelan, J. C. (2001). Conceptualizing stigma. *Annual Review of Sociology, 27*, 363–385.

Activity 7

Many health care providers and consumers now use the Internet to search for health care information. Before going on the Internet, develop a set of questions that you can use to critique the scientific merit of health care information obtained there. List at least five questions in the spaces provided below. (It may be helpful to recall what you have learned about the peer review process that occurs before journal articles are accepted for publication and to review the critiquing criteria in the textbook.)

1.

2.

3.

4.

5.

Activity 8—Web-Based Activity

1. Go to the CINAHL website at https://help.ebsco.com/interfaces/EBSCOhost/training_promotion/Intro_EBSCOhost_Tutorial, and work through the "Introduction to EBSCO*host*" tutorial.

2. Go to the PubMed website at http://www.ncbi.nlm.nih.gov/sites/entrez, and work through the tutorials on PubMed.

Activity 9—Evidence-Informed Practice Activity

1. Use the CINAHL website to do a literature search for the question you developed in Chapter 4.

2. How many articles related to your question did you find?

3. How many of the related articles were research articles?

4. For each article, indicate whether it is a primary or secondary source.

POST-TEST

Select the correct term in brackets to fill in the blanks in the following statements:

a. There are many _____ (advantages; disadvantages) of using computer databases rather than just print databases when doing a literature search.

b. _____ (Primary; Secondary) sources are essential for literature reviews when designing a research proposal.

c. The consumer of research should acquire the ability to _____ (critically evaluate a review of the literature, using critiquing criteria; use primary and secondary sources to write a literature review for a research study).

d. To efficiently retrieve scholarly literature, the nurse must consult both the reference librarian and

_____ (independently use email; use computer CINAHL CD-ROM databases).

Please check with your instructor for the answers to the Post-Test.

REFERENCES

Héon, M., Goulet, C., Garofalo, C., et al. (2016). An intervention to promote breast milk production in mothers of preterm infants. *Western Journal of Nursing Research, 38*(5), 529–552.
Pauly, B., McCall, J., Browne, A. J., et al. (2015). Toward cultural safety: Nurse and patient perceptions of illicit substance use in a hospitalized setting. *Advances in Nursing Science, 38*(2), 121–135.

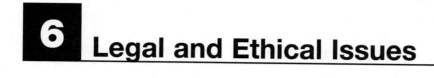

Legal and Ethical Issues

INTRODUCTION

Patient advocacy is one of the primary roles of a professional nurse. Nowhere is this more important than in the field of research. The nurse must be a patient advocate, whether acting as the researcher, a participant in data gathering, a provider of care for research participants, or a research consumer. A multitude of legal and ethical issues exist in research; nurses must be aware of, assess, act on, and evaluate these issues. In addition, nurses need to be knowledgeable about the purpose and functions of the research ethics board (REB) and the federal regulations on which REBs are based.

LEARNING OUTCOMES

On completion of this chapter, you will be able to do the following:
- Describe the historical background that led to the development of ethical guidelines for the use of human participants in research.
- Identify the essential elements of an informed consent form.
- Evaluate the adequacy of an informed consent form.
- Describe the REB's role in the research review process.
- Identify populations of participants who require special legal and ethical research considerations.
- Appreciate the nurse researcher's obligations to conduct and report research in an ethical manner.
- Describe the nurse's role as patient advocate in research situations.
- Discuss the nurse's role in ensuring that Health Canada guidelines for testing of medical devices are followed.
- Discuss animal rights in research situations.
- Critique the ethical aspects of a research study.

Activity 1

Fill in the blanks in the sentences below with the correct terms from the following list (not every term is used):

Anonymity	Justice
Confidentiality	Nursing research committee
Informed consent	Unauthorized research
Research ethics board	Unethical research study

1. A _____ reviews proposals for scientific merit and congruence with the institutional policies and missions.

2. _____ reflects competency standards requiring abstract appreciation of and reasoning about the information provided.

3. _____ exists when the participant's identity cannot be discerned, even by the researcher, from his or her individual responses.

4. A _____ reviews research proposals to ensure protection of the rights of human participants.

5. The idea that human participants should be treated fairly and should not be denied any benefit to which they are entitled is _____.

6. The US Central Intelligence Agency (CIA) funded psychic driving and brainwashing experiments on psychiatric patients in Montreal between 1949 and 1964 (Giniger, 1981). To enhance the psychic driving, increasingly higher levels of electroconvulsive therapy (ECT) were applied to patients as often as three times a day. This treatment would continue for 30 days. There was much damage to patients after such severe treatment. This is considered a(n) _____.

Activity 2

List the three ethical principles that are relevant to the conduct of research involving human participants.

1.

2.

3.

Activity 3

Read the following sample informed consent form, and then review the list of the elements of informed consent that follows the sample. Beside each item on the list, place either a check mark (if the element is included in the consent) or a *0* (if the element is absent from the consent). Summarize your findings at the end of the exercise.

LETTER OF INFORMATION

Open Doors Project

What is the purpose of the study?
You are being invited to participate in a research project entitled "Open Doors." The purpose of this study is to evaluate the effectiveness of a 10-week Peer Advocate Support program in reducing stress and anxiety among post-secondary students at a college in Ontario. The project is anticipated to start in May, 2015 and be completed in May, 2018.

What are you being asked to do in the study?

After reviewing the Letter of Information and agreeing to participate, you will be invited to complete a screening survey. You, if eligible, will be invited to fill out a pre-test survey and a post-test survey following the intervention and 6 months after you have completed the intervention. We will be offering three options for the surveys: (1) paper survey, (2) online survey, and (3) face-to-face interview. These surveys ask questions regarding your background, current and past stressors you may have experienced, the learning conditions in your current program of study, and your sense of well-being. It is estimated that the surveys will take 10 minutes to complete.

Following completion of the screening survey, you, if eligible, will be randomly assigned to one of three study groups:

Peer advocate support: Members of this group will meet with a highly trained nursing student peer advocate for 4–6 hours each week for 10 weeks. The peer advocate will work with the group member to access needed resources and services from their community of residence or the college of enrollment.

Psycho-education group: Members of this group will attend one 15-minute psycho-education group session per week plus self-study for 10 weeks facilitated by a nursing student. Additional activities include self-study for the reminder of the week using a selected anxiety and stress workbook, and use of the log sheet provided in the workbook of the topics you have reviewed and which activities you have completed.

Control group: Members of this group will fill out the pre-test and post-test surveys and will not receive an intervention.

Risks and benefits: Only minimum risks are anticipated for those who take part in this study. However, because the intervention and data-collection procedures ask about lifetime and current stress, it is possible that the recalling of such events may cause some psychological discomforts. If this happens, the peer advocate and data collectors will assess the best course of action based on our safety protocol.

Participating in this research may provide you with the opportunity to improve your stress and anxiety coping skills. In addition, some group members will receive a free anxiety and stress workbook, and all study participants will be entered for a chance to win 1 of 15 Tim Hortons gift cards in the amount of $5.

Confidentiality: All information you provide us during the course of the research project will be held in confidence, and your name will not appear in any report or publication of the research. Your information will be stored in password-protected computers accessible only to the research team in secure offices. Information that you share with us will be stored in this manner for a period of 7 years, then destroyed.

Sharing of study findings: We plan to share this information with research journals and/or peer-reviewed conference presentations. Your information will not be identified in any of these publications or presentations. All data will be kept confidential.

Voluntary participation: Your participation in the study is completely voluntary, and you may choose to stop participating at any time. You don't need to explain why and there is no penalty. If you want to stop participating, you may simply inform the project research assistant and/or peer advocate you are working with.

Withdrawal from the study: You can stop participating in the study at any time, for any reason, if you so decide. Your decision to stop participating or to refuse to answer particular questions will not affect your relationship with the researchers or anyone else involved in the research. Moreover, withdrawal will not affect your status as a student at your college. If you do withdraw from the study and wish to have your information removed from our database, please contact XXX at XXX to make this request.

Answering any questions you may have: If you have questions about this research study, please feel free to contact the project principal investigator XXX, either by telephone at XXX or via email: XXX. This project has been approved by the Research Ethics Board at XXX (education institution). If you have any questions about your rights as a research participant, you can contact Research Ethics Board Chair XXX at XXX.

Sincerely,

Researcher , RN, PhD

Elements of Informed Consent

1. _____ Title of protocol

2. _____ Invitation to participate

3. _____ Basis for participant selection

4. _____ Overall purpose of the study

5. _____ Explanation of benefits

6. _____ Description of risks and discomforts

7. _____ Potential benefits

8. _____ Alternatives to participation

9. _____ Financial obligations

10. _____ Assurance of confidentiality

11. _____ Compensation in case of injury

12. _____ Participant withdrawal

13. _____ Offer to answer questions

14. _____ Concluding consent statement

15. _____ Identification of investigators

Activity 4

The following websites offer comprehensive information about code of ethics and ethical requirements for research:

■ Introductory tutorial for the Tri-Council Policy Statement (TCPS): Ethical Conduct for Research Involving Humans: http://www.pre.ethics.gc.ca/eng/policy-politique/initiatives/tcps2-eptc2/introduction/. The TCPS highlights fundamental ethical issues and principles in research involving human participants. You may consider accessing the online tutorial TCPS 2nd edition: CORE (Course on Research Ethics), available at https://tcps2core.ca/welcome, to complete eight interactive and interesting modules to familiarize yourself with Canada's national standard of ethics for research. You will be awarded a certificate upon completion of the tutorial.

■ Canadian Nurses Association (CNA): https://www.cna-aiic.ca/en/on-the-issues/best-nursing/nursing-ethics. The CNA Nursing Ethics page provides valuable information directly related to nursing ethics. The CNA Code of Ethics for Registered Nurses is a statement of the ethical values of nurses and of nurses' commitments to persons with health care needs and persons receiving care. It is intended for nurses in all contexts and domains of nursing practice and at all levels of decision making.

Nurses must be aware of populations that require special legal and ethical considerations. Review the online resources, and list at least four groups of people who are vulnerable or have diminished autonomy and thus require extra protection as research participants.

1.

2.

3.

4.

Activity 5

Match the two following descriptions of studies with the listed violations of ethical principles. Write the appropriate letters from the list in the blank space that follows each study description. More than one violation may have occurred in the studies; list all violations.

1. The University of California, Los Angeles (UCLA) Schizophrenic Medication Study was a 1983 study examining the effects of withdrawing psychotropic medications from 50 persons who were under treatment for schizophrenia. Twenty-three participants suffered severe relapses after their medications were stopped. The goal of the study was to determine if some schizophrenic persons might do better without medications that had deleterious side effects. Participants were not informed that their symptoms could worsen or about the severity of a potential relapse.

   _____

2. The United States Public Health Service conducted a study from 1932 to 1973 on two groups of African-American male sharecroppers. One group had untreated syphilis; the other did not. Treatment was withheld from the group diagnosed with syphilis, even after the treatment became generally available and was known to be effective. Steps were taken to prevent infected participants from obtaining penicillin. The researchers wanted to study the effects of untreated syphilis.

   _____

   a. The degree of risk outweighed the benefits.
   b. Participants were not informed that they could withdraw from the study at any time.
   c. Participants were not offered or told about the effective treatment that was available.
   d. Informed consent was not obtained.
   e. There was no evidence of REB approval before the start of research.
   f. The participants' right to fair treatment and protection was violated.
   g. Principles of informed consent were violated, or a complete disclosure of potential risk, harm, results, or adverse effects was not made.

Activity 6—Evidence-Informed Practice Activity

This activity assesses the utilization of procedures for protecting basic human rights. Review the articles in Appendices A through D of the text. For each article, describe how informed consent was obtained and whether the author described obtaining permission from the institutional review board.

1. MacDonald, C., Martin-Misener, R., Steenbeek, A., & Browne, A. (2015).

2. Laschinger, H. K. S. (2014).

3. Pauly, B., McCall, J., Browne, A. J., Parker, J., & Mollison, A. (2015).

4. Héon, M., Goulet, C., Garofalo, C., Nuyt, A. M. & Levy, E. (2016).

POST-TEST

1. Researchers and nurses must protect the basic human rights of vulnerable groups. Can research studies be conducted in such populations?

   Yes, because _____

   No, because _____

2. A researcher must receive REB approval (before, after) beginning to conduct research involving humans.

3. When questioning whether a researcher has permission to conduct a study in your hospital, you will want to see documents that verify approval from which group(s)?

   _____

4. Should a researcher list all the possible risks and benefits of participating in a research study even if some people may refuse because these items are listed in detail?

   ☐ Yes   ☐ No

5. If you agreed to collect data for a researcher who had not asked the patient's permission to include that patient in the research study, you would be violating the patient's right to

   _____

6. What are two of the risks of scientific fraud or misconduct?

   _____

   _____

Please check with your instructor for the answers to the Post-Test.

REFERENCES

Giniger, H. (1981, May 16). Montreal hospital pays woman who sued over C.I.A. *The New York Times.* Retrieved from http://query.nytimes.com/gst/fullpage.html?sec=health&res=9802E5D71738F935 A25756C0A967948260

Héon, M., Goulet, C., Garofalo, C., et al. (2016). An intervention to promote breast milk production in mothers of preterm infants. *Western Journal of Nursing Research, 38*(5), 529–552.

Laschinger, H. K. S. (2014). Impact of workplace mistreatment on patient safety risk and nurse-assessed patient outcomes. *Journal of Nursing Administration, 44*(5), 284–290.

MacDonald, C., Martin-Misener, R., Steenbeek, A., et al. (2015). Honouring stories: Mi'kmaq women's experiences with Pap screening in Eastern Canada. *Canadian Journal of Nursing Research, 47*(1), 72–96.

Pauly, B., McCall, J., Browne, A. J., et al. (2015). Toward cultural safety: Nurse and patient perceptions of illicit substance use in a hospitalized setting. *Advances in Nursing Science, 38*(2), 121–135.

7 Introduction to Qualitative Research

INTRODUCTION

The use of scientific methods is important for solving nursing problems. Although knowledge is acquired in a variety of ways, finding optimal ways to answer nursing questions usually entails research. A variety of assumptions and beliefs influence the ways in which nurses see and interpret experiences. One might say that all research is about discovering, coming to know the truth, and gaining knowledge. Historically, most people have viewed science from its empirical perspectives and have placed great value on control, prediction, objectivity, and generalizability (factors discussed later in this book). This perspective takes the view that a single reality exists, and its aim is to identify truth in objective and replicable ways. Empirical studies are essential for investigating particular variables, but they are less helpful for understanding human responses and life experiences.

Whether approaching problems from a quantitative or qualitative standpoint, all researchers are influenced by their personal assumptions and beliefs. Some vigorously argue about the greater worth of one scientific method over another. The quantitative approach to research has been successful in measuring and analyzing data, creating studies that can be replicated, and producing results that can be generalized to other populations. The quantitative method is usually referred to as *empirical analytical research*. Some have argued that qualitative methods are less rigorous than quantitative ones. Others say that because qualitative findings are not generalizable, this research method is less trustworthy. Despite the debate, many now agree that qualitative research is an important method for nursing research because some phenomena or observable events that are of interest to nursing are less easily measured with quantitative methods. Qualitative methods provide another means of gaining nursing knowledge and have become more respected during the last decade.

Qualitative research is a term often applied to naturalistic investigations, or research that involves studying a phenomenon where it occurs. Qualitative research approaches are based on a perceived perspective or holistic world view that recognizes no single reality. Instead, reality is viewed as being based on perceptions that differ from person to person and that change with time; meaning can be truly understood only if it is associated with a specific situation or context. Qualitative research is about understanding phenomena and finding meaning by examining the pieces that make up the whole.

The most common qualitative methods used in nursing research are grounded theory, case study, ethnography, and phenomenology. Each of these methods of investigation presents a unique approach to studying phenomena that are of interest to nurses and nursing.

Evidence-informed practice focuses on findings that come from systematic reviews of the literature that focus on the effectiveness of interventions. As evidence-informed practice becomes more accepted in nursing, old arguments about the place of qualitative research in this process have arisen. Since research designs such as case, descriptive, and evaluative studies continue to be valued less than empirical designs, it is important to understand the contributions made by qualitative research. Questions that are of interest to nursing but have not been previously or thoroughly studied are often best investigated with qualitative methods. When new perspectives are introduced into practice, qualitative investigation may be the best way to gain an early understanding of things that can later be studied with empirical measures. However, reviews of qualitative research on a given topic can also provide insight into practice issues that can be directly applied in clinical settings.

LEARNING OUTCOMES

On completion of this chapter, you will be able to do the following:
- Describe the quantitative research paradigm.
- Describe the beliefs generally held by qualitative researchers.
- Describe the components of a qualitative research report.
- Identify the links between qualitative research and evidence-informed practice.
- Identify four ways qualitative findings can be used in evidence-informed practice.
- Discuss significant issues that arise in conducting qualitative research.

Activity 1—Web-Based Activity

Chapter 7 describes the philosophical foundations of four qualitative methods of research: grounded theory, case study, phenomenology, and ethnography. Although there are other methods of qualitative research, these four are the ones most commonly used in nursing research.

1. Briefly describe each method, and then state its goal or purpose:

   a. Grounded theory

   b. Case study

   c. Phenomenological research

   d. Ethnographic research

2. Choose any search engine, and investigate each of the four methods listed below. It may help to combine each of the terms with the word *nursing*. One or more websites are suggested after each term listed below, but many other sites are available. The goals of this activity are to increase your knowledge about each of these four qualitative research methods, help you differentiate among them, and help you describe how nurses use these research methods.

   List three new things you discover during your Internet exploration about each of these four research methods.

   a. Grounded theory: "Grounded Theory: Doing It as Part of Public Discourse," at https://www. csudh.edu/dearhabermas/grndthry.htm

   b. Case study: "Using Case Study Methodology in Nursing Research," at http://nsuworks.nova.edu/ tqr/vol6/iss2/3/ (Zucker, 2001)

   c. Phenomenology of practice: "Phenomenology of Practice," at http://www.maxvanmanen.com/ phenomenology-of-practice/ (van Manen, 2007); *Nursing Informatics*, at http://nursing-informatics.com/ (Kaminski, 2000–2016)

   d. Ethnography: "Ethnography," at http://en.wikipedia.org/wiki/Ethnography

Activity 2

Complete each sentence in Column A with the appropriate term from Column B. One term is used twice. (For help, review the textbook's glossary.)

Column A

1. _____ explores the lived experience of men who have prostate cancer.

2. _____ uses the past to inform the present.

3. _____ can be on an individual, a group, or an institution.

4. _____ may be followed by empirical study.

5. _____ can generate models of practice.

6. _____ focuses on patterns of behaviour within a culture.

7. _____ evolved from the phenomenological tradition.

Column B

a. Case study

b. Grounded theory

c. Narrative inquiry

d. Ethnographic methods

e. Historical methods

f. Phenomenology

Activity 3

Fill in the blank spaces in the following sentences with the appropriate word or phrase from the text.

1. Qualitative research can also be referred to as _____ research.

2. _____ is the form of data that is gathered for qualitative study.

3. The focus of grounded theory is primarily on dominant _____.

4. Qualitative data are gathered primarily through _____ and _____.

5. Case studies that study cause-and-effect relationships are considered _____ .

6. _____ research reflects on the past to gain understanding to guide the future.

7. _____ developed an ethnographic research method specific to nursing.

Activity 4

Identify which of the four appendices in the text contain studies that are qualitative in nature, and further specify the methodology used in them.

Activity 5—Evidence-Informed Practice Activity

Nurses are under increasing scrutiny from the general public and other professionals over their capacity for compassion. In most cases, assessment of a nurse's level of compassion is used to inform hiring processes. However, compassionate care can be hindered when working in very challenging and high-pressure environments. If a researcher wanted to answer the following question, "What is the process through which nurses come to master working with older adults with dementia while working in high-pressure work environments?" how would he or she go about this?

1. What qualitative method would you use to explore this topic?

2. Why is that method best suited for this purpose?

Activity 6—Web-Based Activity

Unless there is evidence showing that the way we are conducting a particular procedure or continuing a specific protocol is inadequate, most of us assume that if something is being done in nursing practice, it must be correct. Ideas about standards of practice, thoughts about best care, and concerns about quality cause all practitioners to pay greater attention to questions about evidence that does or does not support care decisions. While some nurses have embraced evidence-informed care, others continue to be unsure of its implications and how to provide this form of care. Because most evidence-informed studies focus on quantitative studies (often using clinical trials or intervention studies), less is known about the fit between qualitative research and evidence-informed care.

Read the online article titled "How Can We Argue for Evidence in Nursing?" available at http://www.contemporarynurse.com/archives/vol/11/issue/1/article/1496/how-can-we-argue-for-evidence-in-nursing (Street, 2001). This brief article suggests that decisions nurses make about clinical care are based on the best evidence available. However, many questions about the behavioural aspects of practice still exist. For example, what is it like to be a young woman with type 1 diabetes who has suffered the complications of blindness and kidney failure and spends 3 days a week associating with very ill older individuals who are on dialysis? Think about what that might be like, then consider what evidence you have about how you would best deliver care to this individual if you were the nurse conducting her hemodialysis. What might be known about such care? What might not be known? Although there may be much evidence on care delivery, what in the nursing care delivered to meet the holistic needs of this particular patient could be considered evidence-informed care? What kinds of care might be needed that are different from those for other patients? Qualitative research enables one to investigate questions that are less easily answered through quantitative methods and can provide evidence that can directly affect care delivery.

POST-TEST

1. Which form of qualitative research (indicated by letters in the list below) fits each of the following descriptions?

   A = grounded theory
   B = phenomenology
   C = case study
   D = ethnography

a. _____ This form of research is designed to inductively develop a theory based on observations.

b. _____ This form of research describes patterns of behaviour of people within a culture.

c. _____ Culture is a fundamental value underlying this form of research.

d. _____ This form of research answers questions about meaning.

e. _____ This form of research can help us understand differences and similarities.

2. Choose the correct answer to the following questions:

   A. Which distinction is characteristic of qualitative research methods?
      1. Data are in text form.
      2. Data are dichotomous (either yes or no).
      3. Qualitative research does not generate data.
      4. Data from qualitative studies are inappropriate for analysis.

   B. Which statement is consistent with only qualitative research methods?
      1. The focus of qualitative research is on measuring one or more human characteristics.
      2. The methods are used to attempt to control or eliminate variables that interfere with what is being studied.
      3. The basis for all qualitative interactions is the belief that humans are a composite of many body systems.
      4. The focus of qualitative research methods is the study of human experiences that occur in each person's natural setting.

   C. What should be the determining factor for a researcher to conduct a qualitative study?
      1. The need to test a theory
      2. The nature of the research question
      3. The age and gender of the study participants
      4. The availability of valid instruments to measure the phenomenon

   D. In which instance should a qualitative research design be used instead of a quantitative research design?
      1. When time for data collection is limited
      2. When the research questions are clinical in nature
      3. When the goal is to view the experience in the same way as those who are having the experience
      4. When the researcher is a novice and has minimal experience or skill in scientific problem solving

E. Which aim of research is characteristic of or appropriate for qualitative research methods?
1. Control
2. Prediction
3. Explanation
4. Understanding

F. How are values managed in qualitative research studies compared with how they are managed in quantitative research studies?
1. In both types of study, the goal is to separate values from the research process.
2. In quantitative studies, the values of the researcher are considered study variables.
3. In qualitative studies, the values of the participant are considered an outcome of the study.
4. Although values are acknowledged by both types of research, the quantitative approach uses statistical methods to remove or minimize their impact.

G. Which study purpose is inappropriate for qualitative methods?
1. Testing a new hypothesis
2. Using an intensive approach to data collection
3. Using inductive analysis with the captured data
4. Examining individual responses to an unmodifiable situation

H. What is the purpose of grounded theory research design?
1. To ensure that the theory used has appropriate philosophical underpinnings
2. To move a concept from the perceived view to the received view
3. To test a theory for its specific application
4. To generate a theory from the data collected

I. Which researchers are most associated with the grounded theory research method?
1. Glaser and Strauss
2. Rodgers and Jaycox
3. Watson and Crick
4. Roper and Shapira

J. A nurse studied how older adults used a seniors' centre in Vancouver to access health care. She observed and interviewed a group of 50 older adults and focused on key informants. She also interviewed the centre's social worker, dietitian, and nurse, who were responsible for the program at the centre. Which type of study is this?
1. Phenomenological study
2. Case study
3. Ethnographic study
4. Focus group study

K. The term *triangulation* refers to which of the following?
1. A mathematical technique
2. Combining different methods, theories, data sources, or investigators
3. Information collected becoming repetitive
4. Possible applications of the results of qualitative studies

L. Which specific major premise of grounded theory is represented when the citizens of one nation are outraged when their nation's flag is burned by citizens of another nation? (Select all answers that apply.)
   1. Social interactions are the focus of grounded theory.
   2. Humans act toward objects on the basis of the meaning those objects have for them.
   3. People use interpretive processes to handle and change meanings in dealing with their situations.
   4. Social meanings arise from social interactions with others over time and are embedded socially, culturally, and contextually.

M. How do ethnographic and phenomenological studies differ from one another? (Select all answers that apply.)
   1. Ethnographic studies include both qualitative and quantitative data, whereas phenomenological studies use only qualitative data.
   2. Ethnographic research makes extensive use of case studies, whereas phenomenological research relies more on questionnaires that include multiple-choice questions.
   3. Phenomenological research focuses on the meaning of an event or experience to an individual or group of people; ethnographic research focuses on patterns of behaviour of people within a culture.
   4. Phenomenological research requires that data be collected face-to-face over an extended period of time and that data collection occur in the participant's natural setting; ethnographic studies can be conducted with the researcher and the participant in any setting.

N. Which of the following research questions are most indicative of the phenomenological method? (Select all answers that apply.)
   1. What is the French Canadian lived experience of spirituality?
   2. What is the experience of a recipient of a renal transplant from a living related donor?
   3. What factors influence older adults to seek health care advice following a positive result on a cancer screening examination?
   4. How effective is virtual reality as a method of distraction in reducing chemotherapy-induced distress among teenagers undergoing treatment for cancer?

Please check with your instructor for the answers to the Post-Test.

REFERENCES

Kaminski, J. (2000–2016). *Nursing informatics.* Retrieved from http://nursing-informatics.com/

Street, A. (2001). How can we argue for evidence in nursing? *Contemporary Nurse, 11*(1), 5–8. Retrieved from http://www.contemporarynurse.com/archives/vol/11/issue/1/article/1496/how-can-we-argue-for-evidence-in-nursing

van Manen, M. (2007). *Phenomenology of practice.* Retrieved from http://www.maxvanmanen.com/phenomenology-of-practice/

Zucker, D. (2001). Using case study methodology in nursing research. *The Qualitative Report, 6*(2). Retrieved from http://nsuworks.nova.edu/tqr/vol6/iss2/3/

8 Qualitative Approaches to Research

INTRODUCTION

Qualitative research continues to gain recognition as a sound method for investigating complex human phenomena that are less easily explored with quantitative methods. Qualitative research methods provide ways to address both the science and art of nursing. They are especially well-suited for addressing health and illness phenomena that are of interest to nurses and nursing practice. Nurse researchers and investigators from other disciplines continue to discover the increased value of findings from qualitative studies. Nurses are better prepared to critique the appropriateness of a research design and verify the usefulness of a study's findings when they understand the differences between quantitative and qualitative research approaches.

Although many qualitative research designs might be considered, five methods are most commonly used by nurses: phenomenology, grounded theory, historical research, ethnography, and case study. Community-based participatory research, a newer methodology that is gaining respect from nursing scientists investigating behavioural phenomena, is also described in this chapter. Each qualitative method allows the researcher to approach the phenomena of interest from a different perspective, and each produces findings that address different areas of human experience.

LEARNING OUTCOMES

On completion of this chapter, you will be able to do the following:
- Identify the processes of phenomenological, grounded theory, ethnographic, and case study methods.
- Recognize the appropriate use of historical methods.
- Recognize the appropriate use of community-based participatory research methods.
- Apply critiquing criteria to evaluate a report of qualitative research.

Activity 1

The selection of a qualitative rather than a quantitative design is based on the type of research question asked and the study's purpose. The ability to distinguish the characteristics of qualitative research from those of quantitative research enables the nurse to better understand the way in which a study was conducted and to better interpret its findings. A clear understanding of qualitative research can also help the nurse to better understand how findings from studies can be applied.

1. Complete the following statements related to qualitative research characteristics.

   a. Qualitative research combines the _____ and _____ natures of nursing to better understand the human experience.

b. Qualitative research is used to study human experience and life context in _____
_____.

c. Life context is the matrix of human–environment relationships that emerge over the course of

_____ _____.

d. Qualitative researchers study the _____ _____ of individuals as they carry on their usual activities of daily living, which might occur at home, work, or school.

e. The number of participants in a qualitative study is usually _____ than the number in a quantitative study.

f. Qualitative studies are intended to explore _____ _____ or _____ _____ to better understand the meanings ascribed by individuals living the experience.

g. The choice to use either quantitative or qualitative methods is guided by the _____ _____.

h. One research method is not better than another; the appropriate method is determined when there is a _____ between one's world view, the research question, and the research method.

2. Match the following terms with the appropriate statements.

A. Theoretical sampling	a. _____ Information becomes repetitive
B. Data saturation	b. _____ Select experiences to help the researcher test ideas and gather complete information about developing concepts
C. Qualitative descriptive	c. _____ A research method in which a goal is to change society, collaboratively and following reflection
D. Participatory action research	d. _____ A science whose purpose is to describe particular phenomena, or the appearance of things, as lived experience
E. Case study method	e. _____ The method does not highly abstract the data, but presents it as is
F. Grounded theory method	f. _____ Symbolic categories
G. Phenomenological method	g. _____ Individuals willing to teach the investigator about the phenomenon
H. Secondary sources	h. _____ Provide an in-depth description of the essential dimensions and processes of the phenomenon
I. Domains	i. _____ Provide another perspective of the phenomenon
J. Key informants	j. _____ Inductive approach to develop theory about social processes

3. Your textbook discusses several qualitative research methods in relation to five basic research elements. Read the section in Chapter 8 that describes the research elements for each qualitative method (i.e., identifying the phenomenon, structuring the study, etc.). Briefly describe a key aspect of each element for each qualitative method (see example below). This activity will help you understand the similarities and differences among these methods.

a. Element 1: Identifying the phenomenon

1. Phenomenology (Answer: Focuses on the lived experience of a day-to-day event)

2. Grounded theory

3. Ethnography

4. Historical research

5. Case study

6. Participatory action research

b. Element 2: Structuring the study

1. Phenomenology

2. Grounded theory

3. Ethnography

4. Historical research

5. Case study

6. Participatory action research

c. Element 3: Gathering the data

1. Phenomenology

2. Grounded theory

3. Ethnography

4. Historical research

5. Case study

6. Participatory action research

   d. Element 4: Analyzing the data

      1. Phenomenology

      2. Grounded theory

      3. Ethnography

      4. Historical research

      5. Case study

      6. Participatory action research

   e. Element 5: Describing the findings

      1. Phenomenology

      2. Grounded theory

      3. Ethnography

      4. Historical research

      5. Case study

      6. Participatory action research

Activity 2

Think about an area of clinical practice that is of special interest to you. Consider questions or practice issues related to that clinical area. What kinds of problems might be researched with qualitative perspectives? List two or three topics or problems that could be researched, and choose the most interesting one. Based on the exercise you have just completed on the five elements of research methods, think about the types of qualitative research that would be most appropriate for studying your chosen problem or topic. Select the type of qualitative research you would use, and explain the reasons for your choice.

Activity 3

The five qualitative methods of research are the phenomenological, grounded theory, ethnographic, case study, and historical methods. Using the letters from the key below, indicate which method of qualitative research is described by each statement in the list following the key.

  Key:
  A = Phenomenological
  B = Grounded theory
  C = Ethnographic
  D = Historical
  E = Case study

a. _____ Uses primary and secondary sources

b. _____ Uses emic and etic views of the participants' worlds

c. _____ Research questions are oriented to action or change

d. _____ Central meanings arise from the participants' descriptions of their lived experience

e. _____ Uses theoretical sampling to analyze data

f. _____ Studies the peculiarities and commonalities of a specific case

g. _____ Discovers "domains" to analyze data

h. _____ Provides insight on the past and serves as a guide to the present and future

i. _____ States an individual's history as a dimension of the present

j. _____ Attempts to discover underlying social forces that shape human behaviour

k. _____ Is seldom found in nursing journals

l. _____ Involves interviews with key informants

m. _____ Presents data as a synthesized chronicle

n. _____ Focuses on describing cultural groups

o. _____ Establishes reliability through external and internal criticism

p. _____ Researcher "brackets" personal bias or perspective

q. _____ Can include quantitative data, qualitative data, or both

r. _____ Participants are currently experiencing a circumstance

s. _____ Involves "field work"

t. _____ May use photographs to describe current behavioural practices

u. _____ Uses symbolic interaction as a theoretical base

Activity 4—Evidence-Informed Practice Activity

Critical thinking is an important part of all research. It is important to carefully consider all aspects of the research process before starting research. Keeping the five methods of qualitative research described in the textbook in mind, do the following exercises:

1. Select a qualitative method you found especially interesting. Explain two things about this method that appealed to you.

2. Identify three subject areas for which this method might be helpful in developing nursing knowledge.

    a.

    b.

    c.

3. Choose one of these subject areas, and identify a research question to be studied.

4. Describe the data collection methods you would use for this study.

5. Describe the characteristics of the participants, where you would locate them, how many participants you might include, and the rationale for the number of participants.

6. Briefly explain an important aspect of data analysis using this qualitative method.

7. Describe how you might use the knowledge gained from this study in nursing practice.

Activity 5—Web-Based Activity

Qualitative research is a way to gain knowledge about the complexity of the human health experience in everyday life and over a lifetime. Chapter 8 in your textbook suggests that the use of qualitative research methods can provide evidence to (1) guide nursing practice, (2) contribute to the development of instruments that can be used in quantitative research studies, and (3) develop nursing theory that can guide practice.

On the Internet, access *The Qualitative Report*, at http://nsuworks.nova.edu/tqr/, to see the large number of resources that can increase your understanding of qualitative research and help you better understand how the evidence produced by qualitative research is directly linked to nursing education, clinical practice, and research. Look over a few of these sites. You may want to examine one that is related to a form of qualitative research you have found especially intriguing. It is important that you begin to have some sense of the multitude of work being done using qualitative methods.

After you have finished looking around this web page, click on the following link: http://www.groundedtheoryonline.com/ to the "Grounded Theory Online" web page. On the top, click on "What is Grounded Theory?" Read through this information and answer the following questions:

a. What is theoretical sensitivity?

b. How is research conducted using this method?

c. How does the data analysis proceed? How is this process different from other qualitative data analysis methods?

POST-TEST

For questions 1 through 5, answer true *(T)* or false *(F)*.

1. _____ Qualitative research focuses on the whole of human experience in naturalistic settings.

2. _____ "External criticism" in historical research refers to the authenticity of data sources.

3. _____ In qualitative research studies, the number of participants is as great as that usually found in quantitative studies.

4. _____ The researcher is viewed as the major instrument for data collection.

5. _____ Qualitative studies strive to eliminate extraneous variables.

For questions 6 through 14, select the best answer.

6. In qualitative research, to what does the term *saturation* refer?
   a. Data repetition
   b. Participant exhaustion
   c. Researcher exhaustion
   d. Sample size

7. In qualitative research, data are often collected by which of the following procedures?
   a. Questionnaires sent out to participants
   b. Observation of participants in their natural settings
   c. Interviews
   d. All of the above

8. The qualitative method that uses symbolic interaction as the theoretical base for research is known as which of the following?
   a. Phenomenology
   b. Grounded theory
   c. Ethnography
   d. Historical research

9. Which qualitative method attempts to construct the meaning of the lived experience of human phenomena?
   a. Phenomenology
   b. Grounded theory
   c. Ethnography
   d. Historical research
   e. Case study
   f. Community-based participatory research

10. Which qualitative research method is the most appropriate for answering the question, "What changes in nursing practice occurred after the outbreak of SARS in Canada?"
    a. Phenomenology
    b. Grounded theory
    c. Ethnography
    d. Historical research
    e. Case study
    f. Community-based participatory research

11. Which qualitative research method would be most appropriate for studying the effect of culture on the health behaviours of urban Aboriginal youth?
    a. Phenomenology
    b. Grounded theory
    c. Ethnography
    d. Historical research
    e. Case study
    f. Community-based participatory research

12. Which qualitative method would be most appropriate for studying a family's experience with cystic fibrosis?
    a. Phenomenology
    b. Grounded theory
    c. Ethnography
    d. Historical research
    e. Case study
    f. Community-based participatory research

13. Which qualitative method would you use to study the spread of human immunodeficiency virus infection/acquired immune deficiency syndrome (HIV/AIDS) in an urban area?
    a. Phenomenology
    b. Grounded theory
    c. Ethnography
    d. Historical research
    e. Case study
    f. Community-based participatory research

14. Which data analysis process is not used with grounded theory methodology?
    a. Bracketing
    b. Axial coding
    c. Theoretical sampling
    d. Open coding

Please check with your instructor for the answers to the Post-Test.

9 Introduction to Quantitative Research

INTRODUCTION

The term *research design* is used to describe the overall plan of a particular study. The research design is the researcher's plan for answering specific research questions in the most accurate and efficient way. In quantitative research, this plan outlines how hypotheses will be tested. The design ties together the present research problem, knowledge of the past, and implications for the future. Thus, the choice of design reflects the researcher's experience, expertise, knowledge, and biases.

LEARNING OUTCOMES

On completion of this chapter, you will be able to do the following:
- Define research design.
- Identify the purpose of the research design.
- Define control as it affects the research design.
- Compare and contrast the elements that affect control.
- Begin to evaluate the degree of control that should be exercised in the design.
- Define internal validity.
- Identify the threats to internal validity.
- Define external validity.
- Identify the conditions that affect external validity.
- Identify the links between study design and evidence-informed practice.
- Evaluate the design by using the critiquing questions.

Activity 1

Match the definitions in Column A with the research design terms in Column B. Each term is used only once, and not all terms are used. Check the textbook glossary for help with terms.

Column A

1. _____ A sample of participants who are similar to one another

2. _____ Participants' responses being studied

3. _____ Methods to keep study conditions constant during the study

4. _____ Consideration of whether the study is possible and practical

5. _____ Vehicle for testing hypotheses or answering research questions

6. _____ Process to ensure every participant has an equal chance of being selected

7. _____ Degree to which a research study is consistent within itself

8. _____ Degree to which the study's results can be applied to the larger population

9. _____ All parts of a study follow logically from the problem statement

Column B

a. External validity

b. Internal validity

c. Accuracy

d. Research design

e. Control

f. Random sampling

g. Feasibility

h. Homogeneous sampling

i. Objectivity

j. Reactivity

Activity 2

For each abstract presented below, identify the potential threats to internal validity from the following list. Explain why it is a problem, and suggest how this problem can be corrected.

History	Mortality
Instrumentation	Selection bias
Maturation	Testing

1. A study investigated the efficacy of an additional medication administration web course in increasing nursing students' self-evaluated competence on medication administration. Nursing students self-evaluated their medication administration competence before ($n = 244$) and after ($n = 192$) the web-based medication course. An online self-evaluation questionnaire was developed to measure students' competence on basic pharmacotherapy, intravenous medication and infusion, blood transfusion, and epidural medication. (Mettiäinen, Luojus, Salminen, et al., 2014)

2. The aim of this study was to describe undergraduate nurses' perceptions of spirituality/spiritual care and their perceived competence in delivering spiritual care. Questionnaires were completed by a convenience sample of 618 undergraduate nurses from 6 universities in 4 European countries in 2010. (Ross, van Leeuwen, Baldacchino, et al., 2014)

3. This study prospectively monitored study burnout for a national sample of nursing students during their upper years in their nursing program and at follow-up 1 year post-graduation. Changes in mean burnout scores as measured by the Oldenburg Burnout Inventory across time were estimated using data collected form a cohort of nursing students surveyed at four points in time over 4 years: Three times during the final 2 years of nursing school and 1 year post-graduation. A sample of 1,702 respondents was prospectively followed from late autumn 2002 to spring 2006. (Rudman & Gustavsson, 2012)

4. A large randomized controlled trial of an intervention for disadvantaged male youth grades 7–10 was conducted in high-crime Chicago neighborhoods. The intervention was delivered by two local non-profits and included regular interactions with a prosocial adult, after-school programming, and in-school programming designed to reduce common judgement and decision-making problems related to automatic behaviour and biased beliefs, or what psychologists call cognitive-behavioural therapy (CBT). We randomly assigned 2,740 youth to programming or to a control group. About 50% of those offered programming participated, with the average participant attending 13 sessions. (Heller, Pollack, Ander, et al., 2013)

5. Under conditions of typical clinical practice, this study examined whether outcomes achieved with brief counselling from prenatal care providers and a self-help booklet could be improved by adding more resource-intensive cognitive-behavioral programs. 390 English-speaking women 18 years of age or older who self-reported to be active smokers at their initial prenatal appointment took part in the study. Participants were randomized to one of three groups: (1) a self-help booklet tailored to smoking patterns, stage of change, and lifestyle of pregnant smokers; (2) the booklet plus access to a computerized telephone cessation program based on interactive voice response technology; or (3) the booklet plus proactive telephone counseling from nurse educators using motivational interviewing techniques and strategies. No attempt was made to change smoking-related usual care advice from prenatal providers. Biochemically confirmed abstinence was measured by level of

cotinine in urine samples obtained during a routine prenatal visit at approximately the 34th week of pregnancy. 22% of participants were confirmed as abstinent with no significant differences found between intervention groups. (Ershoff, Quinn, Boyd, et al., 1999)

Activity 3

The term *research design* denotes the overall plan for answering research questions, including the method and specific plans to control other factors that could influence the results of the study. To become acquainted with the major elements of the design of a study, read the article by Pauly, McCall, Browne, et al. (2015) (Appendix C), and answer the following questions:

a. What was the setting for the study?

b. Who were the participants?

c. How was the sample selected?

d. What information is missing?

e. Was this a homogeneous sample?

f. How were variables measured and constancy maintained?

g. Which group served as the control group?

Activity 4

The critical appraisal of the research design requires that the research consumer address seven important questions:

1. Is the type of study design employed appropriate?

2. Does the researcher use the various concepts of control that are consistent with the type of design chosen?

3. Does the design seem to reflect the issues of feasibility?

4. Does the design flow from the proposed research question, theoretical framework, literature review, and hypothesis?

5. What were the threats to internal validity, and how did the investigators control for each?

6. What were the threats to external validity, and how did the investigators control for each?

7. Is the design appropriately linked to the levels of evidence hierarchy?

Use the critiquing criteria from Chapter 9 to critique the research design of the study described in the article by Laschinger (2014) in Appendix B of the text. Explain your answers.

   a. Is the design appropriate?

   b. Is the control consistent with the research design?

   c. Think about the feasibility of this study. Is this a study that would be expected of a master's student in nursing? Of a doctoral student? Explain the reasoning behind your answer.

   d. Does the design logically flow from the problem, framework, literature review, and hypothesis?

   e. What were the threats to internal validity, and how did the investigators control for each?

   f. What were the threats to external validity, and how did the investigators control for each?

Activity 5—Evidence-Informed Practice Activity

Review Figure 3-1 from your textbook, reproduced below. For each level of evidence, indicate on the list following the figure whether the evidence is *(A)* expert opinion, *(B)* qualitative, *(C)* quantitative, *(D)* a combination of qualitative and quantitative, or *(E)* anecdotal.

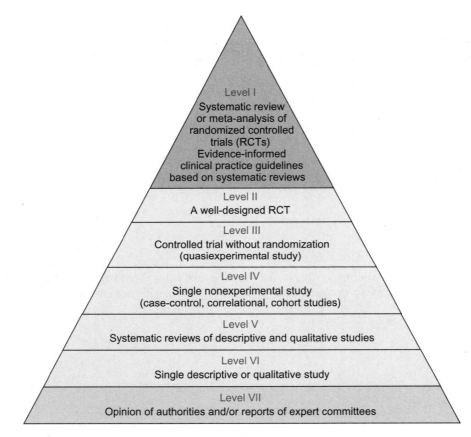

Levels of Evidence

Evidence hierarchy for rating levels of evidence, associated with a study's design. Evidence is assessed at a level according to its source. Based on Melynk, B. M., & Finoult-Overholt, E. (2011). *Evidence-based practice in nursing & literature: A guide to best practice* (2nd ed.). Philadelphia: Lippincott, Williams and Wilkins.

1. Level I:

2. Level II:

3. Level III:

4. Level IV:

5. Level V:

6. Level VI:

7. Level VII:

Activity 6—Web-Based Activity

Use Google Scholar or your library to locate the following article:

  Samuels-Dennis, J. A., Ford-Gilboe, M., & Ray, S. (2011). Single mothers' adverse and traumatic experiences and post-traumatic stress symptoms. *Journal of Family Violence, 26*(1), 9–20.

1. Briefly assess the major components of the research design.

   a. In your own words, what was the purpose of the study?

   b. What was the setting for the study?

   c. Who were the participants?

   d. How was the sample selected?

   e. What was the research treatment?

   f. How did the researchers attempt to control elements affecting the results of the study?

POST-TEST

1. Fill in the blanks in the sentences below by selecting from the following list of terms. Not all terms will be used.

constancy	mortality
control	internal validity
feasibility	external validity
selection bias	accuracy
reliability	history
maturation	

   a. _____ is used to hold steady the conditions of the study.

   b. _____ is used to indicate that all aspects of a study logically follow from the problem statement.

   c. The believability of a study in terms of the world in general is known as _____.

   d. The developmental, biological, or psychological processes known as _____ operate in a person over time and may influence the results of a study.

   e. Time, participant availability, equipment, money, experience, and ethics are factors influencing the _____ of a study.

   f. Selection bias, mortality, maturation, instrumentation, testing, and history influence the _____ of a study.

   g. Voluntary (rather than random) assignment to an experimental or control condition creates a situation known as _____.

Please check with your instructor for the answers to the Post-Test.

REFERENCES

Ershoff, D. H., Quinn, V. P., Boyd, N. R., et al. (1999). The Kaiser Permanente prenatal smoking-cessation trial: When more isn't better, what is enough? *American Journal of Preventive Medicine*, *17*(3), 161–168.

Heller, S., Pollack, H. A., Ander, R., et al. (2013). Preventing youth violence and dropout: A randomized field experiment (No. w19014). National Bureau of Economic Research.

Mettiäinen, S., Luojus, K., Salminen, S., et al. (2014). Web course on medication administration strengthens nursing students' competence prior to graduation. *Nurse Education in Practice*, *14*(4), 368–373.

Ross, L., van Leeuwen, R., Baldacchino, D., et al. (2014). Student nurses perceptions of spirituality and competence in delivering spiritual care: A European pilot study. *Nurse Education Today*, *34*(5), 697–702.

Rudman, A., & Gustavsson, J. P. (2012). Burnout during nursing education predicts lower occupational preparedness and future clinical performance: A longitudinal study. *International Journal of Nursing Studies*, *49*(8), 988–1001.

Samuels-Dennis, J. A., Ford-Gilboe, M., & Ray, S. (2011). Single mothers' adverse and traumatic experiences and post-traumatic stress symptoms. *Journal of Family Violence, 26*(1), 9–20.

10 Experimental and Quasiexperimental Designs

INTRODUCTION

This chapter contains exercises for two types of design: experimental and quasiexperimental. These types of design allow researchers to test the effects of nursing actions and make statements about cause-and-effect relationships. Therefore, they can be helpful in testing solutions to nursing practice problems. However, a researcher chooses the design that allows a given situation or problem to be studied in the most accurate and effective way. Thus, not all problems are amenable to immediate study by these two types of design. Rather, the choice of design depends on the development of knowledge relevant to the problem as well as the researcher's knowledge, experience, expertise, preferences, and resources.

LEARNING OUTCOMES

On completion of this chapter, you will be able to do the following:
- List the criteria necessary for inferring cause-and-effect relationships.
- Distinguish the differences between experimental and quasiexperimental designs.
- Define problems with internal validity that are associated with experimental and quasiexperimental designs.
- Describe the use of experimental and quasiexperimental designs for evaluation research.
- Critically evaluate the findings of selected studies in which cause-and-effect relationships were tested.
- Apply levels of evidence to experimental and quasiexperimental designs.

Activity 1

Fill in the blank spaces in each of the descriptions below with a term selected from the following list of types of experimental and quasiexperimental designs. Each term is used only once. Consult the textbook glossary for definitions of the terms.

> after-only experiment
> after-only nonequivalent control group
> experimental
> true experiment
> nonequivalent control group
> Solomon four-group
> time series

1. _____ designs are particularly suitable for testing cause-and-effect relationships because they help eliminate potential alternative explanations (threats to validity) for the findings.

2. The type of design that has two groups identical to the true experimental design plus an experimental after-group and a control after-group is known as a(n) _____ design.

3. A research approach used when only one group is available to study for trends over a longer period is called a(n) _____ design.

4. The _____ design is also known as the post-test-only control group design, in which neither the experimental group nor the control group is pretested.

5. If a researcher wanted to compare the results obtained from an experimental group with those obtained from a control group but was unable to conduct pretests or randomly assign participants to groups, the study would be known as a(n) _____ design.

6. The _____ design includes three properties: randomization, control, and manipulation.

7. When participants cannot be randomly assigned to experimental and control groups but can be pretested and post-tested, the design is known as a(n) _____ design.

Activity 2

A large hospital's education department wants to test a program for educating its nurses about pain management and changing their attitudes to pain, using a questionnaire that measures the nurses' knowledge and attitudes about pain. Your responsibility is to design a study to examine the outcome of this program.

1. You decide to use a Solomon four-group design. Put an X in the appropriate blank space in the chart below to indicate which of the four groups are to receive the pretest and post-test pain questionnaire and which groups are to participate in the experimental teaching program.

Group	Pretest Questionnaire	Teaching Program	Post-Test Questionnaire
Group A	_____	_____	_____
Group B	_____	_____	_____
Group C	_____	_____	_____
Group D	_____	_____	_____

2. How would you assign nurses to each of the four groups?

3. What would you use as a pretest (for groups receiving the pretest)?

4. What is the experimental treatment?

5. What is the outcome measure for each group?

6. According to your reading, for what types of issues is this design particularly effective?

7. What is the major advantage of this type of design?

8. What is a disadvantage of this type of design?

Activity 3

Answer the questions that follow the descriptions of experimental and quasiexperimental studies given below.

1. The purpose of this study was to examine caregiver outcomes in 14 programs. Caregiver outcomes in regard to the following were measured: burden, quality of life, perceived health, opinion on institutionalization (just prior to patient admission, and at 2 weeks, 2 months, and 6 months after admission), and satisfaction with the program at three points after patient admission (Warren, Ross-Kerr, Smith, et al., 2003).

   a. What type of design was used?

   b. Why is this a reasonable choice of design?

2. The purpose of this study was to evaluate the effectiveness of interventions provided by a community mental health team in reducing stress in caregivers for persons with dementia. Following an initial multidisciplinary assessment, all caregivers of those with dementia were invited to participate; 26 caregivers consented and participated in all stages of data collection. Data were collected with the Caregiver Strain Index at initial assessment and again at 3 and 6 months (Hoskins, Coleman, & McNeely, 2005).

   a. What type of design was used?

   b. What are the advantages of this design?

   c. What are the disadvantages of this design?

Activity 4

1. Both experimental and quasiexperimental designs are important in nursing research to guide evidence-informed practice.

   a. In what circumstances might it be advantageous to use an experimental design?

   b. In what circumstances might it be advantageous to use a quasiexperimental design?

2. What must the researcher do to generalize the findings of a quasiexperimental research study?

3. What must a clinician do before applying research findings to practice?

Activity 5—Web-Based Activity

In this activity, you are looking for experimental nursing research studies.

1. Go to https://www.ncbi.nlm.nih.gov/pubmed/ and type "experimental studies nursing" into the search bar. Look at the top of the list of items. How many articles have been found?

2. Find the article by Irvine, Billow, Bourgeois, and Seeley (2012), "Mental illness training for long term care staff." Is this an actual experimental study? If not, what is it?

3. Now click on "Customize" under "Article types" near the left top. From the drop-down menu, select "Randomized Controlled Trial" and then click on "Show" at the bottom. After this, click on "Randomized Controlled Trial" under "Article types." How many articles were found with this limit?

4. Go to the article by Bastani, Hashemi, Bastani, and Haghani (2010), "Impact of preconception health education on health locus of control and self-efficacy in women."

   a. What type of design is used in this study?

   b. How is randomization applied?

   c. What do the authors say about the limitation of the study?

   d. Are the findings of this study generalizable to a larger population of interest? If not, why not?

Activity 6—Evidence-Informed Practice Activity

When using evidence-informed practice strategies, the first step is to decide which level of evidence a research article provides. Review Figure 3-1 (reproduced below) from your textbook, and then do the exercises that follow it.

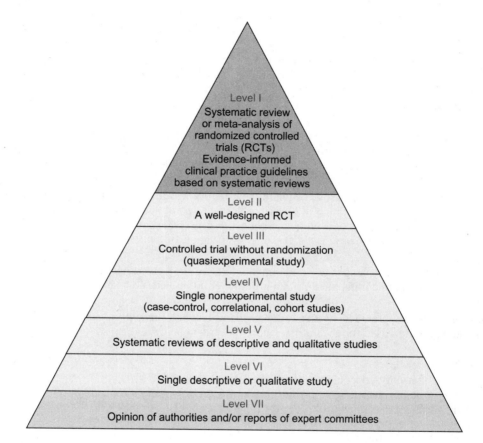

Levels of Evidence

Evidence hierarchy for rating levels of evidence associated with a study's design. Evidence is assessed at a level according to its source. Based on Melynk, B. M., & Finoult-Overholt, E. (2011). *Evidence-based practice in nursing & literature: A guide to best practice* (2nd ed.). Philadelphia: Lippincott, Williams and Wilkins.

1. Review the article by Laschinger (2014) in Appendix B of the textbook and select the appropriate level of evidence for that study.

2. Review the study by Pauly, McCall, Browne, et al. (2015) in Appendix C of the text and select the appropriate level of evidence for that study.

POST-TEST

1. Indicate whether the following studies are experimental *(E)*, or quasiexperimental *(Q)*.

   a. _____ Fifty teenaged mothers are randomly assigned to an experimental parenting support group or a regular support group. Before and at the end of the 3-month program, mother–child interaction patterns in the two groups are compared.

   b. _____ Patients on separate units are given a questionnaire on their satisfaction with care to fill out at the end of their first hospital day and on the day of discharge. The patients on one unit receive care directed by a nurse case manager, and those on the other unit receive care from the usual rotation of nurses. Patient satisfaction scores are compared.

   c. _____ Students are randomly assigned to two groups. One group receives an experimental independent study program, and the other receives the usual classroom instruction. Both groups receive the same post-test to evaluate learning.

   d. _____ A study is conducted to compare the effectiveness of a music relaxation program with that of silent relaxation in lowering blood pressure. Participants are randomly assigned to groups, and blood pressure is measured before, during, and immediately after the relaxation exercises.

   e. _____ Reading and language development skills are compared between a group of children with chronic otitis media and a group of children with no history of ear problems.

2. Using the numbers provided by the following key, indicate the type of experimental or quasi-experimental design used for each of the studies described below.

   Key: 1 = After-only
   2 = After-only nonequivalent control group
   3 = True experiment
   4 = Nonequivalent control group
   5 = Time series
   6 = Solomon four-group

   a. _____ Nurses are randomly assigned to a new self-study program or to the usual electrocardiography teaching program. Both groups' knowledge of electrocardiography is tested before and after the program.

   b. _____ Babies with positive results on toxicology screening tests at birth are randomly assigned into groups receiving either routine care or care under a special public health nurse intervention program. Health outcomes are assessed and compared at 6 months.

   c. _____ Health care outcomes from a school with a new school nurse clinic are assessed at the end of 1 year and compared with health outcomes at a comparable school that does not have a clinic.

d. _____ Diabetic patients are randomly assigned either to one of two control groups receiving routine home health care or to one of two groups participating in a new diabetes education program. Patients in one of the control groups and in one of the teaching groups are tested on their knowledge of diabetes as soon as they are assigned to a group. Patients in the other two groups are not pretested. All patients complete a post-test at the conclusion of the 3-week program.

e. _____ A high school implements a peer program for preventing acquired immune deficiency syndrome (AIDS). Students of a high school without the program serve as a control group. A test assessing the students' knowledge of AIDS is administered at both schools before and after the program is completed.

f. _____ Trends in patient falls are summarized each week, 1 year before implementation of a new hospital-based quality assurance program, and for the first year after implementation.

Please check with your instructor for the answers to the Post-Test.

REFERENCES

Bastani, F., Hashemi, S., Bastani, N., et al. (2010). Impact of preconception health education on health locus of control and self-efficacy in women. *Eastern Mediterranean Health Journal, 16*(4), 396–401.

Hoskins, S., Coleman, M., & McNeely, D. (2005). Stress in careers of individuals with dementia and community mental health teams: An uncontrolled evaluation study. *Journal of Advanced Nursing, 50*(3), 325–333.

Irvine, A. B., Billow, M. B., Bourgeois, M., et al. (2012). Mental illness training for long term care staff. *Journal of the American Medical Directors Association, 13*(1), 81.e7–81.e13.

Laschinger, H. K. S. (2014). Impact of workplace mistreatment on patient safety risk and nurse-assessed patient outcomes. *Journal of Nursing Administration, 44*(5), 284–290.

Pauly, B., McCall, J., Browne, A. J., et al. (2015). Toward cultural safety: Nurse and patient perceptions of illicit substance use in a hospitalized setting. *Advances in Nursing Science, 38*(2), 121–135.

Warren, S., Ross-Kerr, J., Smith, D., et al. (2003). The impact of adult day programs on family caregivers of elderly relatives. *Journal of Community Health Nursing, 20*(4), 209–221.

11 Nonexperimental Designs

INTRODUCTION

Nonexperimental designs can provide large amounts of data that can help fill in the gaps in nursing research. These designs help us to clarify information, see the real world, and assess relationships between variables, and they can provide clues for future and more controlled research. Experimental, quasiexperimental, and nonexperimental designs complement each other; each provides components necessary for our knowledge base. Nonexperimental designs enable us to discover some of the territory of nursing knowledge before we try to rearrange parts of it. They can be the base on which knowledge is built and then further refined with quasiexperimental and experimental research.

LEARNING OUTCOMES

On completion of this chapter, you will be able to do the following:
- Describe the overall purpose of nonexperimental designs.
- Describe the characteristics of survey and relationship or difference designs.
- Define the differences between survey and relationship or difference designs.
- List the advantages and disadvantages of surveys and each type of relationship or difference design.
- Identify methodological, secondary analysis, and meta-analysis research.
- Identify the purposes of methodological, secondary analysis, and meta-analysis research.
- Discuss relational inferences versus causal inferences as they relate to nonexperimental designs.
- Identify the criteria used to critique nonexperimental research designs.
- Apply the critiquing criteria to the evaluation of nonexperimental research designs as they appear in research reports.
- Apply levels of evidence to nonexperimental designs.

Activity 1

After each of the sentences below the word puzzle, fill in the blank space with the appropriate word or words (some will be used more than once). Then find and circle each of those words in the puzzle. The words are printed in a straight line, but they may read up or down; left to right; right to left; or diagonally. Any single letter may be used in more than one word. There are no spaces or hyphens between words; thus, a multiword answer will appear as a single word.

Experimental Design Puzzle

```
L  O  N  G  I  T  U  D  I  N  A  L  D  M  E
C  I  S  P  U  E  Q  W  H  X  O  I  Y  H  X
C  R  F  L  G  Y  Q  E  R  C  X  E  C  G  P
U  W  O  L  Z  S  B  Q  F  H  V  O  H  H  O
N  T  L  S  C  I  S  Z  A  R  R  O  I  U  S
L  G  T  R  S  D  L  D  U  R  Z  L  D  O  T
U  E  I  O  I  S  Q  S  E  D  L  V  W  O  F
I  U  W  S  J  J  E  L  O  S  Y  U  H  I  A
G  T  D  K  X  O  A  C  I  E  M  D  I  I  C
Q  W  R  E  E  T  O  K  T  T  E  S  T  A  T
A  S  A  M  I  K  E  N  B  I  B  H  U  L  O
D  U  O  O  K  L  H  N  P  H  O  B  Z  V  F
M  C  N  G  U  L  U  E  O  L  Y  N  R  K  C
K  A  M  F  G  U  P  Q  S  B  Z  L  A  H  T
L  W  J  F  V  N  E  W  J  S  W  L  E  L  V
```

1. This type of design is known more for the breadth of data collected than for the depth of its data. _____

2. A major disadvantage of this design is the length of time needed for data collection. _____

3. The main question is whether or not variables covary. _____

4. These words mean "after the fact." _____

5. Eliminates the confounding variable of maturation. _____

6. Quantifies the magnitude and direction of a relationship. _____

7. Collects data from the same group at several points in time. _____

8. This can be surprisingly accurate if the sample is representative. _____

9. Uses data from one point in time. _____

10. Based on two or more naturally occurring groups with different conditions of the presumed independent variable. _____

Activity 2

Below the following table are descriptions of the advantages and disadvantages of various types of nonexperimental designs. For each type of design listed in the table, pick at least one advantage and one disadvantage that accurately describe a quality of that design. Then insert their number codes (e.g., A1, D2) in the appropriate spaces in the table.

	Advantages	Disadvantages
Correlational	_____	_____
Cross-sectional	_____	_____
Ex post facto	_____	_____
Longitudinal	_____	_____
Prospective	_____	_____
Retrospective	_____	_____
Survey	_____	_____

Advantages

A1 A great deal of information can be obtained economically from a large population.
A2 Has the ability to assess changes in the variables of interest over time
A3 Explores the relationship between variables that are inherently not manipulable
A4 Offers a higher level of control than a correlational study
A5 Each participant is followed separately and serves as his or her own control.
A6 Stronger than a retrospective study because of the degree of control of extraneous variables
A7 Less time-consuming and less expensive; thus, more manageable for the researcher

Disadvantages

D1 Does not allow one to draw a causal linkage between two variables
D2 An alternative hypothesis could be the reason for the relationships.
D3 The researcher is unable to manipulate the variables of interest.
D4 The researcher is unable to determine a causal relationship between variables owing to lack of manipulation, control, and randomization.
D5 The information obtained tends to be superficial.
D6 The researcher must know sampling techniques, questionnaire construction, interviewing, and data analysis.
D7 No randomization in sampling because the study involves only pre-existing groups
D8 Internal validity threats (such as testing and mortality) are present.
D9 Participant loss to follow-up and attrition may lead to unintended sample bias that affects external validity and generalizability of findings.

Activity 3

Following the list below are excerpts from abstracts of several nonexperimental studies. Select the type of design used for each study from the list. Not every design is used in the study examples, and some designs are used more than once.

correlation study
cross-sectional
ex post facto
longitudinal
methodological
meta-analysis
prospective
retrospective
survey comparative
survey descriptive
survey exploratory

(n.b.: Some studies use more than one type of nonexperimental design.)

1. The study investigated the efficacy of a medication administration web course in increasing nursing students' self-evaluated competence on medication administration. Finnish nursing students self-evaluated their medication administration competence before and after the web-based medication course. 244 students answered the questionnaire before and 192 after the web course. (Mettiäinen, Luojus, Salminen, et al., 2014)

Types of design:

_____

2. The study aims to describe undergraduate nurses'/midwives' perceptions of spirituality/spiritual care and their perceived competence in delivering spiritual care, and to test the proposed method and suitability of measures for a larger multinational follow-up study. The research team administered questionnaires completed by a sample of 618 undergraduate nurses/midwives from six universities in four European countries in 2010. (Ross, van Leeuwen, Baldacchino, et al., 2014)

Types of design:

_____

3. This study prospectively monitored Swedish nursing students' burnout during the upper years of their nursing program and 1 year post-graduation. Data were collected at four points in time over 4 years: three times during higher education and 1 year post-graduation. A longitudinal sample of 1,702 respondents was prospectively followed from late autumn 2002 to spring 2006. (Rudman & Gustavsson, 2012)

Types of design:

_____

4. This study examined responses to a survey on violence in the workplace from a sample of 8,780 registered nurses practicing in 210 hospitals in the Canadian provinces of Alberta and British Columbia. Findings relate to the frequency of violence against nurses, reported as the number of times they experienced a violent incident in the workplace. Multiple regression modelling using the individual nurse as the unit of analysis showed the significant predictors of emotional abuse to be age, casual job status, quality of care, and degree of hospital restructuring. Using the hospital as the unit of analysis the predictors were found to be quality of care, age, relationships with hospital staff, presence of violence prevention measures, and province. (Duncan, Hyndman, Estabrooks, et al., 2001)

Types of design:

_____

5. This study estimated the effectiveness of problem-based learning in developing nursing students' critical thinking skills. Nine articles representing eight randomized controlled trials were included in the analysis. The pooled effect size showed problem-based learning was able to improve nursing students' critical thinking, compared with traditional lectures. (Kong, Qin, Zhou, et al., 2014)

Types of design:

_____

Activity 4

Use the critiquing criteria described in the textbook to analyze the following excerpt from a study.

In a 1997 article by Mohr, the objective was as follows: "This study is the context portion of a larger study that described the experience of 30 nurses in Texas, USA, who worked in for-profit psychiatric hospitals during a documented period of corporate deviance. The objective of the contextual portion was to describe the major findings in 1991–1992 of investigating agencies that probed the scandal" (p. 39). The sample consisted of over 1,240 pages and 40 hours of corporate records obtained under subpoena, and written and oral testimony before the U.S. House Select Committee on Children, Youth, and Families.

1. What type of research design was used?

The findings fell under four themes: insurance games, dumping of patients, patient abuse, and playing with the language.

The conclusion, "Organizational deviance may become more widespread in profit-driven systems of care. Lobbying for whistleblower protection, collective advocacy, and creative educational reforms are used" is presented at the start of the article. However, under the "Discussion and Recommendations" section, the author states, "As suggested by social scientists, research can serve as the basis for reflection, critique, and action. . . . For example, because nurses are professionals who have a special contract with the public and are concerned with health teaching and promotion, they might implement counterhegemonic activity by collective advocacy and criticizing information distortion."

2. Does the research go beyond the relational parameters of the findings and erroneously infer cause-and-effect relationships between the variables? (Circle the correct answer and explain your choice.)

Yes   No

Explanation:

Activity 5

Review the "Critical Thinking Decision Path: Nonexperimental Design Choices" found in the textbook. If you wanted to test a relationship between two variables in the past—such as the incidence of reported back injuries among nurses working in newborn nurseries compared with that of nurses working in long-term care—which design would you use?

Activity 6—Web-Based Activity

This activity will help you find nursing research survey instruments if you are considering gathering data for a nonexperimental survey study. Use two search engines (Google and Google Scholar) and one website (PubMed) to find instruments; then compare the three sources to determine which is the most helpful to you.

Upon reviewing the results you have obtained from PubMed, Google, and Google Scholar, answer the following four questions for each source.

a. How many results were identified?

b. Print the first page, and review the first five citations. Do these citations contain information about survey instruments that are available for use in nursing research?

c. How is the information presented? Is it presented in a manner that is useful for planning research?

d. How current is the information?

1. First, go to the National Library of Medicine PubMed site at http://www.ncbi.nlm.nih.gov/pubmed. At the top left, make sure that "PubMed" appears in the window, or select it from the drop-down menu. In the search bar to the right, type in "Nursing Research Survey Instruments" and click on "Search." Review the results you obtain and answer questions a through d.

2. Now go to the Google website at http://www.google.ca. In the box, type in "Nursing Research Survey Instruments." Click on "Google Search." Review the results you obtain and answer questions a through d.

3. Now go to the Google Scholar website at http://scholar.google.com. In the box, type "Nursing Research Survey Instruments." Click on "Search." Review the results you obtain and answer questions a through d.

Activity 7—Evidence-Informed Practice Activity

Select the best response to each of the following questions.

1. What is the value of nonexperimental studies, such as those that demonstrate a strong relationship in predictive correlational studies for evidence-informed practice?

   a. They have no value.

   b. They provide evidence only for training purposes.

   c. They demonstrate cause-and-effect relationships and can be used in decision making regarding changes in practice.

   d. They lend support for attempting to influence the independent variable in a future intervention study.

2. Which of the following nonexperimental designs provides a stronger quality of evidence for evidence-informed practice than the other designs because the researcher can determine the problem's incidence and its possible causes?

   a. Cross-sectional

   b. Longitudinal cohort

   c. Survey

3. When you, as a research consumer, are using the evidence-informed practice model to consider a change in practice, you will initially base your decision on the strength and quality of evidence provided by the meta-analysis. What other characteristics are important for you to consider? (There are two correct answers.)

   a. Clinical expertise

   b. Client values

   c. The strength of the evidence

   d. The quality of the evidence

   e. The literature review

POST-TEST

Choose from among the words in the following list to complete this test. Each word will be used at least once but some will appear in more than one answer.

comparative	exploratory	methodological	survey
correlational	ex post facto	prospective	variables
cross-sectional	interrelational	relationship-difference	
descriptive	longitudinal	retrospective	

1. In comparative surveys, the researcher does not manipulate the _____ but assesses data to provide information for future nursing intervention studies.

2. _____ is the broadest category of nonexperimental design.

3. The category identified in item 2 can be further classified as _____ and _____.

4. According to this textbook, the second major category of nonexperimental design includes _____ studies.

5. When examining the relationship between two or more variables, the researcher is using _____ design.

6. _____ designs have many similarities to quasi-experimental designs.

7. _____ design used in epidemiological work is similar to ex post facto design.

8. Your textbook discusses the following three types of developmental studies:

   a.

   b.

   c.

9. _____ studies involve collecting data at one point in time whereas _____ studies involve collecting data from the same group at different points in time.

10. A(n) _____ study looks at presumed causes and moves forward in time to presumed effects.

11. When a researcher is trying to link present events to past events, he or she is using a _____ design.

12. The _____ researcher is interested in identifying an intangible construct (concept) and making it tangible, with a paper-and-pencil instrument or observation protocol.

Please check with your instructor for the answers to the Post-Test.

REFERENCES

Duncan, S. M., Hyndman, K., Estabrooks, C. A., et al. (2001). Nurses' experience of violence in Alberta and British Columbia hospitals. *Canadian Journal of Nursing Research Archive*, *32*(4), 57–78.

Ershoff, D. H., Quinn, V. P., Boyd, N. R., et al. (1999). The Kaiser Permanente Prenatal Smoking-Cessation Trial: When more isn't better, what is enough? *American Journal of Preventive Medicine*, *17*(3), 161–168.

Heller, S., Pollack, H. A., Ander, R., et al. (2013). *Preventing youth violence and dropout: A randomized field experiment* (Working Paper No. 19014). National Bureau of Economic Research. Retrieved from http://www.nber.org/papers/w19014

Kong, L. N., Qin, B., Zhou, Y. Q., et al. (2014). The effectiveness of problem-based learning on development of nursing students' critical thinking: A systematic review and meta-analysis. *International Journal of Nursing Studies*, *51*(3), 458–469.

Mettiäinen, S., Luojus, K., Salminen, S., et al. (2014). Web course on medication administration strengthens nursing students' competence prior to graduation. *Nurse Education in Practice*, *14*(4), 368–373.

Mohr, W. K. (1997). Outcomes of corporate greed. *Image: The Journal of Nursing Scholarship*, *29*(1), 39–45.

Ross, L., van Leeuwen, R., Baldacchino, D., et al. (2014). Student nurses perceptions of spirituality and competence in delivering spiritual care: A European pilot study. *Nurse Education Today*, *34*(5), 697–702.

Rudman, A., & Gustavsson, J. P. (2012). Burnout during nursing education predicts lower occupational preparedness and future clinical performance: A longitudinal study. *International Journal of Nursing Studies*, *49*(8), 988–1001.

12 Sampling

INTRODUCTION

Sampling is a process of selection in which individuals, objects, animals, or events are chosen to represent the population of a study. The ideal sampling strategy enables the researcher to choose a sample that represents the target population and controls for bias as much as possible to ensure that the research will be valid. The specific research question (or questions) determines the selection of the sample, the variables to measure, and the sampling frame. Real-world factors regarding efficiency, practicality, ethics, and the availability of participants can affect the ideal strategy for a given study.

LEARNING OUTCOMES

On completion of this chapter, you should be able to do the following:
- Identify the purpose of sampling.
- Define population, sample, and sampling.
- Compare a population and a sample.
- Discuss the eligibility criteria for sample selection.
- Define nonprobability and probability sampling.
- Identify the types of strategies for both nonprobability and probability sampling.
- Identify the types of qualitative sampling.
- Compare the advantages and disadvantages of specific nonprobability and probability sampling strategies.
- Discuss the contribution of nonprobability and probability sampling strategies to the strength of evidence provided by study findings.
- Discuss the factors that influence determination of sample size.
- Discuss the procedure for drawing a sample.
- Identify the criteria for critiquing a sampling plan.
- Use the critiquing criteria to evaluate the "Sample" section of a research report.

Activity 1

Match the category of sampling with each of the following sampling strategies. (In the blank spaces, write P for probability sampling and N for nonprobability sampling.)

1. _____ Convenience sampling

2. _____ Purposive sampling

3. _____Simple random sampling

4. _____ Quota sampling

5. _____ Cluster sampling

6. _____ Systematic sampling

7. _____ Stratified random sampling

Activity 2

From the following list, select the sampling strategy used for each of the study samples described below the list. In the space preceding each sample description, write the letter that corresponds to the strategy. Refer to the textbook glossary for definitions of terms.

  a. Convenience sampling
  b. Quota sampling
  c. Purposive sampling
  d. Simple random sampling
  e. Stratified random sampling
  f. Systematic sampling

1. _____ The sample for a study of critical thinking behaviour among undergraduate nursing students consisted of students enrolled in junior- and senior-level courses in three schools of nursing. In each program, students were invited to participate until a total sample representing 10% of the junior-level students and 10% of the senior-level students was achieved.

2. _____ Every eighth person on a diabetic clinic patient roster was asked to participate in the study. A random number table was used to start the sampling during the first sampling interval.

3. _____ Using a random number table, a sample of 50 participants was selected from a list of all mothers who gave birth in the county during the first 6 months of the year.

4. _____ A sample selected from residents of eight nursing homes in Alberta consisted of cognitively impaired persons with no physical impairments or other psychiatric illnesses.

5. _____ The sample consisted of parents chosen because of their knowledge and experience of being a parent with a child in a neonatal intensive care unit (NICU). Inclusion criteria for parents were (1) a child admitted to the NICU for more than a week, (2) a gestation at birth of 26 or more weeks, (3) a child on a ventilator for at least 3 days, and (4) a child discharged home within the previous 6 months.

6. _____ The sample consisted of adolescent mothers meeting the eligibility requirements and recruited from referrals to the community health services division of the public health department. Selection continued until the sample reached the target number of 144 participants. A computer-based procedure randomly assigned the mothers to one of two groups.

7. _____ For a study on educational opportunities for nurses in various ethnic groups, a list of all the nurses in Ontario was sorted by ethnicity. The sample consisted of 10% of the nurses in each ethnic group, selected according to a table of random numbers.

8. _____ A total of 155 infants were enrolled and divided into an intervention group of 72 infants and a control group of 83 infants. The numerical assignment was based on weight and gestational age.

Activity 3

1. Refer to the study by Laschinger (2014) in Appendix B of the textbook.

   a. Is the sample adequately described?

   ☐ Yes   ☐ No

   b. Do the sample characteristics correspond to the larger population?

   ☐ Yes   ☐ No   ☐ Maybe

   c. What sampling strategy was used in this study?

   d. Is this a probability or nonprobability sample?

   e. Is the sample size appropriate?

   ☐ Yes   ☐ No   ☐ Unsure

2. List one advantage of using the sampling strategy described in this study.

3. List one disadvantage of using the sampling strategy described in this study.

4. How does this sampling strategy support evidence in nursing practice?

Activity 4

Using the Critical Thinking Decision Path in Chapter 12 in the textbook, indicate whether the following statements are true or false.

1. _____ Nonprobability sampling is associated with less generalizability to the larger population.

2. _____ Convenience sampling limits the generalizability of findings largely because of the self-selection of participants.

3. _____ Nonprobability sampling strategies are more time consuming than probability strategies.

4. _____ Random sampling has the greatest risk of bias and is moderately representative.

5. _____ The easier the sampling strategy, the greater the risk of bias, and as sampling becomes easier to implement, the risks of bias and limited representation of the population increase.

6. _____ Of the sampling strategies listed, purposive sampling procedures are the least generalizable.

7. _____ Stratified random sampling uses a random selection procedure for obtaining sample participants.

Activity 5

The critical appraisal of the sampling strategy for a quantitative article requires that the following questions be addressed:

1. Have the sample characteristics been completely described?

2. Can the parameters of the study population be inferred from the description of the sample?

3. To what extent is the sample representative of the population as defined?

4. Are criteria for eligibility in the sample specifically identified?

5. Have sample delimitations been established?

6. Would it be possible to replicate the study sample?

7. How was the sample selected? Is the method of sample selection appropriate?

8. What kind of bias, if any, is introduced by this method?

9. Is the sample size appropriate? How is it substantiated?

10. Are there indications that the rights of the participants have been ensured?

11. Do the researchers identify the limitations in the generalizability of the findings from the sample to the population? Are the limitations appropriate?

12. Do the researchers indicate how replication of the study with other samples would provide increased support for the findings?

Review the following excerpt from the study by Samuels-Dennis, Xia, Secord, et al. (2016). Using the critiquing criteria from Chapter 12 listed above, and the questions that follow the excerpt, critique the sampling process used in this study.

A sample of community residents (N = 240) was randomly allocated to four groups. Group 1 served as a control group and received *usual care* provided by primary care practitioners at the community health centre. Group 2 received 10 weeks (2–3 hours/week) of case management and health advocacy support delivered by highly trained nursing students (health advocate). Health advocates assisted participants with the development of life/health goals and worked with them to access the services/resources needed to address those goals. Additionally, a major emphasis of the health advocates' role was to identify gaps in service delivery (e.g., absent or poor quality service) and to use a variety of strategies to ensure that the community either helps improve the accessibility and quality of existing services or puts in place nonexistent services/resources. The efficacy of this component of HAP [Health Advocacy Project] has previously been demonstrated by Dr. Sullivan, the co-lead of a study that examined women exiting domestic violence shelters in the U.S. (Bybee & Sullivan, 2002). Group 3 received 10 weeks (1–2 hours/week) of evidence-based mental health care delivered by a CNS [clinical nurse specialist]. CNS care is grounded in the findings of theoretical and empirical works previously completed by the project lead. Specifically, CNS activities included advanced case management, evidence-informed treatment modalities for MDD [major depressive disorder] and PTSD [posttraumatic stress disorder] and interpersonal counseling. Group 4 received the combined services of the health advocate and CNS.

This study used a longitudinal randomized control trial (RCT) design. Participants were recruited via posters, traditional and nontraditional media, community agency referrals, and word of mouth. Self-referring participants were prescreened using computer-assisted personal interviewing (CAPI) to determine their eligibility. Eligible participants were randomly assigned to one of four study groups using a randomization table that accounts for sex (male, female) and diagnosis (MDD, PTSD). Randomization table was generated by the study statistician. Community residents were approached for participation if they meet the following criteria: (a) male or female age 16 to 65 years; having an income below the low-income cut-off (LICO) for their household size; and (b) currently experiencing PTSD or depression. Individuals with a current substance abuse addiction, severe mental illness such as schizophrenia, and/or who reported current suicidal ideations were excluded. Excluded individuals were provided with contact information for various community agencies based on need.

The study protocol was reviewed and approved by each institutional research ethics board. Eligible participants who consented to partake in the study were asked to complete the registration form and the baseline survey questionnaire. Follow-up data were collected via face-to-face or telephone contact by a research assistant, blinded to group assignment, immediately after the intervention was completed and 6 months, 12 months, and 18 months following the completion of the intervention.

This was a randomized control trial, the gold standard to determine effectiveness. There were, however, two limitations. First, it is possible that the community population may have possessed a stress profile that was significantly different from that of the vulnerable groups whom we wished to generalize our findings. A post-hoc analysis was incorporated to ascertain this effect. Second, because this study was being undertaken in a community environment, some participants may take part in other concurrent community-based campaigns that may also influence the study outcomes. We have incorporated questions about community resources access that assisted us with assessing for these effects. Despite the aforementioned limitations, the findings from the current study will be helpful to validate the effectiveness of the health advocacy role in improving depressive and anxiety symptoms among low-income youth and adults seeking mental health care in Ontario communities.

This study is considered timely because it will help us to build a body of knowledge that addresses the responsive provision of trauma-informed mental health care using traditional and nontraditional roles. It also has the potential to help researchers and clinicians identify the elements of the types of care and the places/spaces within low-income community that currently lack the high-quality services needed to promote the mental health of youth and adults who reside there. Working collaboratively with York University, the study has developed a knowledge translation plan to communicate study findings and key learnings to municipal and community leader partners to generate awareness and interest in transferring the project to all of Ontario and potentially Canada.

1. Have the sample characteristics been completely described?

2. Can the parameters of the study population be inferred from the description of the sample?

3. To what extent is the sample representative of the population defined?

4. Are criteria for eligibility in the sample specifically identified?

5. Have sample delimitations been established? (Explain your answer.)

6. Would it be possible to replicate the study sample? (Explain your answer.)

7. How was the sample selected? Is the method of sample selection appropriate?

8. What kind of bias, if any, is introduced by this method?

9. Is the sample size appropriate? How is it substantiated?

10. Are there indications that the rights of the participants have been ensured?

11. Do the researchers identify the limitations in the generalizability of the findings from the sample to the population? Are the limitations appropriate?

12. Do the researchers indicate how replication of the study with other samples would provide increased support for the findings?

Activity 6—Web-Based Activity

The text defines *evidence-informed practice* (EIP) as the integration of best research evidence with clinical expertise and patient values. EIP enables nurses to use research findings to make decisions to improve practice. Teams of nurses apply numerous study findings to improve outcomes of practice with individuals, families, and other health care providers. This has led to more effective patient teaching and higher-quality care.

The Registered Nurses' Association of Ontario (RNAO) has created a library of best practice guidelines (BPG), found at http://rnao.ca/bpg. Spend some time perusing the available BPG on the website and select those that suit your practice interests. Review the five Evidence-Informed Practice Tips in Chapter 12 before answering the following questions:

What is the relationship between sampling and EIP decision making? In other words, how will the sampling strategy in a meta-analysis of study like a BPG influence how you and your colleagues make decisions about changing the practice in your health care setting?

POST-TEST

Fill in the blank spaces to complete the sentences below.

1. A statistical technique known as _____ may be used to determine sample size in quantitative studies.

2. _____ is a subset of all units (i.e., items or people) forming a population from which a sample will be chosen.

3. _____ sampling is the use of the most readily accessible persons or objects as participants in a study.

4. The advantages of _____ sampling are low bias and maximal representativeness, but the disadvantage is the labour in drawing a sample.

5. A(n) _____ can be used to select an unbiased sample or an unbiased assignment of participants to treatment groups.

6. A(n) _____ sample is one whose key characteristics closely approximate those of the population.

7. _____ is a small sample study conducted as a prelude to a larger-scale (parent) study.

8. Types of nonprobability sampling include _____, _____ _____, and _____ sampling.

9. Successive random sampling of units that progress from large to small and meet sample eligibility criteria is known as _____ sampling.

10. In certain qualitative studies, participants are added to the sample until _____ occurs (i.e., new data no longer emerge during data collection).

Please check with your instructor for the answers to the Post-Test.

REFERENCES

Bybee, D. I., & Sullivan, C. M. (2002). The process through which an advocacy intervention resulted in positive change for battered women over time. *American Journal of Community Psychology*, *30*(1), 103–132.

Laschinger, H. K. S. (2014). Impact of workplace mistreatment on patient safety risk and nurse-assessed patient outcomes. *Journal of Nursing Administration, 44*(5), 284–290.

Samuels-Dennis, J., Xia, L., Secord, S., et al. (2016). Health Advocacy Project: Evaluating the benefits of service learning to nursing students and low income individuals involved in a community-based mental health promotion project. *International Journal of Nursing Education Scholarship, 13*(1). doi: 10.1515/ijnes-2015-0069

13 Data-Collection Methods

INTRODUCTION

> Observe, probe
> Details unfold
> Let nature's secrets
> Be stammeringly retold.
> —Goethe

Consumers of research need the skills to evaluate and critique data-collection methods in published research studies. In developing these skills, it is helpful to have an appreciation of the process used or of the critical-thinking "journey" that the researcher made, to be ready to collect the data. Each of the preceding chapters presented an important preliminary step in the planning and designing phases before data collection. And while most researchers are eager to begin collecting data, the planning beforehand for data collection is very important. Planning includes identifying and prioritizing data needs, developing or selecting the appropriate data-collection tools, and selecting and training data-collection personnel.

The five data-collection methods differ in their basic approaches and have different strengths and weaknesses. Be prepared to question the appropriateness of the measures chosen by the researcher to gather data about the variable of concern. This includes determining the objectivity, consistency, quantifiability, extent of observer intervention, and obtrusiveness of the chosen data-collection method.

LEARNING OUTCOMES

On completion of this chapter, you will be able to do the following:
- Define the types of data-collection methods used in nursing research.
- List the advantages and disadvantages of each of these methods.
- Compare how specific data-collection methods contribute to the strength of evidence in a research study.
- Critically evaluate the data-collection methods used in published nursing research studies.

Activity 1—Evidence-Information Practice Activity

Review each of the articles cited below. Be especially thorough in reading the sections that relate to data-collection methods. Answer the questions that follow each of the citations below. For some questions, there may be more than one answer.

Study 1

MacDonald, Martin-Misener, Steenbeek, et al. (2015) (in Appendix A of the textbook)

1. Which of the following data-collection methods was/were used in this research study?
   a. A physiological measure
   b. An observational measure
   c. An interview measure
   d. A questionnaire
   e. Records of available data

2. What was the rationale for the appropriateness of the data collection method(s)?

3. What is your opinion of the success of the method(s) chosen?

Study 2

Laschinger (2014) (in Appendix B of the textbook)

1. Which of the following data-collection methods was/were used in this research study?
   a. A physiological measure
   b. An observational measure
   c. An interview measure
   d. A questionnaire
   e. Records of available data

2. What was the rationale for the appropriateness of the data-collection method(s)?

3. What is your opinion of the success of the method(s) chosen?

Study 3

Pauly, McCall, Browne, Parker, et al. (2015) (in Appendix C of the textbook)

1. Which of the following data-collection methods was/were used in this research study?
   a. A physiological measure
   b. An observational measure
   c. An interview measure
   d. A questionnaire
   e. Records of available data

2. What were the strengths of the chosen method(s)?

Study 4
Héon, Goulet, Garofalo, Nuyt, et al. (2016) (in Appendix D of the textbook)

1. Which of the following data-collection methods was/were used in this research study?
    a. A physiological measure
    b. An observational measure
    c. An interview measure
    d. A questionnaire
    e. Records of available data

2. What was the rationale for the appropriateness of the data collection method(s)?

3. What is your opinion of the success of the method(s) chosen?

Activity 2
With help from Chapter 13 of the textbook, fill in the spaces in the following statements with the correct words, and then circle those words in the puzzle below.

1. Baccalaureate-prepared nurses are _____ of research.

2. _____ methods use technical instruments to collect data about a patient's physical, chemical, microbiological, or anatomical status.

3. _____ is the distortion of data as a result of the observer's presence.

4. _____ are best used when a large response rate and an unbiased sample are important.

5. Data collection with _____ is subject to problems of availability, authenticity, and accuracy.

6. _____ measurements are especially useful when there are a finite number of questions to be asked and the questions are clear and specific.

7. Essential in the critique of data-collection methods is the emphasis on the appropriateness, _____, and _____ of the method used.

8. _____ raises ethical questions (especially issues of informed consent); therefore, it is not often used in nursing.

9. _____ is the consistency of observations between two or more observers.

10. _____ is the process of translating concepts or variables into measurable phenomena.

11. The _____ is a format that uses closed-ended items, and there are a fixed number of alternative responses.

12. _____ is the method for objective, systematic, and quantitative descriptions of communications and documentary evidence.

13. This exercise is supposed to be _____!

```
D E L I V E R S T A T I S T C S Y E S P A S
S S A C A B I N E T F O R K A Z O S P E I O
I A W O P E R A T I O N A L I Z A T I O N B
G T S N O R N E V E R B Y D N E A U X B T J
N S Y S T E M A T I C A J H T B S D V S E E
I F L I K E R T S C A L E E R R O Y A E R C
F A K S C A L E S N O V N O C A A U L R R T
H C U T A C R A T I M A P V E T P U I V A I
Y T B E B H I R T E M A H V W K I C D A T V
P C O N T E N T A N A L Y S I S P V O T E I
R O Y C B K D S I S R T S A D V A N E I R T
E R E Y O D U G K A T P I B I O I G O R Y
A V S I B R Q U E S T I O N N A I R E N E C
C I A R E S E A R C H L L R E A C E S O L O
T O B M E X C E L A E O O D A T A C O V I N
I U E A E V A L I D S T G N O S T O O E A S
V N Y E S S I N T E R V I E W S A R F R B U
I H A P P I E N E S S P C A T A G D U N I M
T X C I T E D E L P H I A T O T P S N V L E
Y C E A T U B B S A N D L D O N N M A R I R
Y A B L E A C O N C E A L M E N T O O T T S
A I K E V A L I K E I I A B C O N S U M Y S
```

Activity 3

You are reviewing a study, and concealment is necessary; there is no other way to collect the data, and the data collected will not have negative consequences for participants.

1. Name at least one population in which concealment is not uncommon.

2. How would you obtain the participants' consent?

3. What is the major reason for concealment?

Activity 4

You are asked to participate in discussions about impending research in your community. The purpose of the study is to identify the health status, beliefs, practices, current preventive services, and accessibility and availability of health services in your rural community. Describe what you would consider in the selection of a data-collection method. Review each method, discuss the pros and cons of choosing a specific data-collection method, and state the rationale for your final selection. What would be your thoughts concerning instruments and types?

Activity 5

Refer to Chapter 13 in the textbook, and circle the letter before the correct answer to each of the following questions. Some questions will have more than one correct answer.

1. What is the primary advantage of physiological measures?
   a. The measuring tool never affects the phenomena being measured.
   b. They are among the easiest types of methods to implement.
   c. It is unlikely that study participants can distort physiological information.
   d. They are objective, sensitive, and precise.
   e. All of the above

2. Self-report measures are usually more useful than observation measures in obtaining information about which of the following?
   a. Socially unacceptable or private behaviours
   b. Complex research situations in which it is difficult to separate processes and interactions
   c. Situations in which the researcher is interested in character traits
   d. All of the above

3. Which of the following would be considered the disadvantages of using observational data collection methods?
   a. Individual bias may interfere with data collection.
   b. Ethical concerns may become increasingly significant.
   c. Individual judgements and values influence observers' perceptions.
   d. All of the above

4. In nursing research, when might questionnaires be an appropriate method for data collection?
   a. Whenever expense is a concern for the researcher
   b. When a researcher is interested in obtaining information directly from the participants
   c. When the researcher needs to collect data from a large group of participants who are not easily accessed
   d. When accuracy is of the utmost importance to the researcher

5. Which of the following is an advantage of using existing records or available data to answer a research question?
   a. The use of available data reduces the risk of researcher bias in data collection.
   b. The time needed for the research study can be reduced.
   c. The consistent collection of information over time allows the researcher to study trends.
   d. All of the above

Activity 6—Web-Based Activity

Numerous evidence-informed projects are being undertaken in the nursing field. This online resource *Evidence-Based Practice Building Blocks: Comprehensive Strategies, Tools, and Tips* is available at https://uihc.org/evidence-based-practice-building-blocks-comprehensive-strategies-tools-and-tips at the University of Iowa. Click on "View a sample" and review the guidebook to promote your understanding and adoption of evidence-informed practices.

POST-TEST

Read each question thoroughly, and then circle the correct answer from the list below.

1. What term denotes the process of translating concepts into observable and measurable phenomena?
   a. Objectivism
   b. Systematization
   c. Subjectivism
   d. Operationalization

2. Research questions about psychosocial variables can be best answered by using which data-gathering technique(s)?
   a. Observation
   b. Interviews
   c. Questionnaires
   d. All of the above

3. Which of the following terms denotes the collection of data from each participant in the same or a similar manner?
   a. Repetition
   b. Dualism
   c. Consistency
   d. Recidivism

4. Which of the following terms denotes the consistency of observations between two or more observers?
   a. Intrarater reliability
   b. Interrater reliability
   c. Consistency reliability
   d. Repetitive reliability

5. Physiological and biological measurements might be used by nurse researchers when studying which of the following variables? (Select all that apply.)
   a. A comparison of student nurses' ACT scores and grade point averages (GPAs)
   b. Hypertensive patients' responses to a stress test
   c. Children's dietary patterns
   d. The degree of pain relief achieved after guided imagery

6. Scientific observations should fulfill which of the following conditions?
   a. Observations are consistent with the study objectives.
   b. Observations are standardized and systematically recorded.
   c. Observations are checked and controlled.
   d. All of the above

7. In a research study, a participant observer spent regularly scheduled hours at a shelter for homeless people and occasionally stayed overnight. The people staying in the home were told that this person was conducting a research study. The researcher freely engaged in conversation and openly observed these homeless individuals. What was the observational role of the researcher?
   a. Concealment without intervention
   b. Concealment with intervention
   c. No concealment without intervention
   d. No concealment with intervention

8. In unstructured observation, which of the following might occur? (Select all that apply.)
   a. Extensive field notes are recorded.
   b. Participants are told what behaviours are being observed.
   c. The researcher frequently records interesting anecdotes.
   d. All of the above

9. Which of the following is inconsistent with a Likert scale?
   a. It contains closed-ended items.
   b. It contains open-ended items.
   c. It contains lists of statements.
   d. Items are evaluated on the amount of agreement.

10. Although it is acceptable to use numerous instruments in a research study, the study is more acceptable if only one method is used for data collection.

    Is the above statement true or false?
    a. True
    b. False

11. Social desirability is seldom a concern for researchers when interviewing is the data-collection method used in the study.

    Is the above statement true or false?
    a. True
    b. False

12. A researcher wants to use a questionnaire in a study but cannot find one that will gather the desired information about a particular variable. The decision is made to develop a new instrument. Which of the following should the researcher do?
    a. Define the construct, formulate the items, and assess the items for content validity.
    b. Develop instructions for users, and pilot the instrument.
    c. Estimate reliability and validity.
    d. All of the above

13. The researcher who invests significant time developing an instrument has a professional responsibility to publish the results.

    Is the above statement true or false?
    a. True
    b. False

14. To evaluate the adequacy of various data-collection methods, which of the following should be observed in the written research report?
    a. Clear identification of the rationale for selecting a physiological measure
    b. Observational measures that address the problems of bias and reactivity
    c. Clear explanation of how interviews were conducted and how interviewers were trained
    d. All of the above

15. In conducting a research study, the researcher has a responsibility to ensure that all study participants receive the same information and that data are collected from all participants in the same manner.

    Is the above statement true or false?
    a. True
    b. False

Please check with your instructor for the answers to the Post-Test.

REFERENCES

Héon, M., Goulet, C., Garofalo C., et al. (2016). An intervention to promote breast milk production in mothers of preterm infants. *Western Journal of Nursing Research, 385*(5), 529–552.

Laschinger, H. K. S. (2014) Impact of workplace mistreatment on patient safety risk and nurse-assessed patient outcomes. *Journal of Nursing Administration, 44*(5), 284–290.

Macdonald, C., Martin-Misener, R., Steenbeek, A., et al. (2015). Honouring stories: Mi'kmaq women's experiences with Pap screening in Eastern Canada. *Canadian Journal of Nursing Research, 47*(1), 72–96.

Pauly, B., McCall, J., Browne, A. J., et al. (2015). Toward cultural safety: Nurse and patient perceptions of illicit substance use in a hospitalized setting. *Advances in Nursing Science, 38*(2), 121–135.

14 Rigour in Research

INTRODUCTION

If a friend tells you, "Hey, I found a new restaurant that you will really love," you will consider that information from at least two perspectives before you spend your money there. First, does this person know what she is talking about when it comes to your taste in food? Second, has this person given you good information about food in the past?

You answer "no" to the first question. You prefer seafood served in an elegant setting, and your friend prefers pizza served in a place with sawdust on the floor. Knowing this, you will consider her opinion to be invalid for you. You will never give this restaurant another thought.

But if you answer "yes" to the first question because you and your friend share similar tastes in food, you will move on to the second question. You remember the tough fettuccini, the superb Southern fried chicken, the undercooked pizza, and the "hockey puck" biscuits from earlier recommendations. It is likely that while you and your friend share food preferences, her information is unreliable. You cannot trust her to give you good information. If you are feeling like having an adventure, you may try the new restaurant.

The validity and reliability of the data collection instruments used in a study should be regarded in the same way as a friend's advice about restaurants. Is the instrument valid? Does it provide accurate information? Is this information trustworthy? Is the instrument reliable? Does it provide consistent information whenever it is used? Consideration of both validity and reliability influences your confidence in the results of the study.

LEARNING OUTCOMES

On completion of this chapter, you will be able to do the following:
- Discuss the purposes of reliability and validity.
- Define reliability.
- Discuss the concepts of stability, equivalence, and homogeneity as they relate to reliability.
- Compare the estimates of reliability.
- Define validity.
- Compare content validity, criterion-related validity, and construct validity.
- Discuss how measurement error can affect the outcomes of a research study.
- Identify the criteria for critiquing the reliability and validity of measurement tools.
- Use the critiquing criteria to evaluate the reliability and validity of measurement tools.
- Discuss the purpose of credibility, auditability, and fittingness.
- Define credibility.
- Define auditability.
- Define fittingness.
- Apply the critiquing criteria to evaluate the rigour in a qualitative report.
- Discuss how evidence related to research rigour contributes to clinical decision making.

Activity 1

Either random error *(R)* or systematic error *(S)* may occur in a research study. For each of the following examples, identify the type of measurement error, and describe how the error might be corrected.

1. _____ The scale used to measure daily weights was inaccurate, reading 1500 g less than the actual weight.

    Correction:

2. _____ Students chose the socially acceptable responses on an instrument for assessing attitudes toward people with acquired immune deficiency syndrome (AIDS).

    Correction:

3. _____ The evaluators were confused about how to score wound healing.

    Correction:

4. _____ The subjects were nervous about taking the psychological tests.

    Correction:

Activity 2

Validity is the extent to which an instrument measures what it is intended to measure. Fill in the blank spaces in the sentences below (ratings from panels of experts) with the appropriate terms from the following list.

concurrent validity	content validity	contrasted groups
construct validity	convergent validity	criterion-related validity
divergent validity	face validity	factor analysis
hypothesis testing	content experts	predictive validity

1. "_____ was supported by exploratory factor analysis and item-scale correlation. Factor analysis yielded the three subscales of consistent use, correct use, and communication. In

   addition, _____ was supported in that subscales allowed investigators to differentiate between consistent and non-consistent condom users. Cronbach's alpha coefficient rated between .749 and .884 for the subscales, and .96 for the overall scale." (Zhao, Wong, Miu, et al., 2016)

2. _____ is an intuitive, preliminary type of instrument evaluation.

3. "In a study, the investigators developed a self-assessment Clinical Competency Questionnaire for

   upcoming baccalaureate nursing graduates. To test _____ the researchers first conducted focus groups with clinical instructors to establish a list of possible competencies needed for upcoming baccalaureate nursing students. Subsequently, they asked a panel of three faculty experts to review the specifications of the selected items and judge the degree of item significance to student competencies required for their first year of practice." (Liou & Ching, 2014)

4. Construct validity, an assessment of the relationship between the instrument and the

   underlying theory, can be measured in several ways. List three of these: _____, _____, and _____.

5. "A Nursing Students' Knowledge and Attitudes of LGBT Health Concerns (NKALH) survey (Cornelius & Carrick, 2008) was developed to address pertinent LGBT health care issues. Content for the instrument was based on two surveys that examined medical students' knowledge, attitudes, and skills (Kelley, Chou, Dibble, et al., 2008) and ability to care for LGBT patients (Sanchez, Rabatin, Sanchez, et al., 2006). The survey was examined by content experts (nurses and health educators) knowledgeable about LGBT health care who recommended revisions to several questions. Next, it was piloted with three nursing students, who were able to complete the survey

   in 10 to 15 minutes (Cornelius & Carrick, 2008)." Both processes added _____ and _____ to the survey.

6. "Previous studies have demonstrated that the Daily Hassles for Adolescents Inventory has good _____, as evidenced by its significant relationship to adjustment measures." (Wright, Creed, & Zimmer-Gembeck, 2010)

7. "A 2-week test–retest of 67 registered nurses of the original 374 [RNs] yielded an alpha of .97. Six nursing experts were therefore invited to assess the instrument for _____. The experts were asked to rate the degree of relevance of each item using a four-point scale (1 point was "not relevant"; 2 points, "somewhat relevant"; 3 points, "relevant but needs minor revision"; and 4 points, "very relevant") and to comment on item clarity, simplicity, and/or ambiguity." (Sirisawasd, Chaiear, Johns, et al., 2014)

Activity 3

An instrument is considered reliable if it is accurate and consistent. If the concept being studied is stable, the same results should occur when the measurement is repeated.

1. Identify three concepts that are related to reliability.

    1. _____

    2. _____

    3. _____

2. Give an example of each of the two types of tests for stability.

    1. _____

    2. _____

3. In what instance would it be better to use an alternative validity/reliability assessment rather than a test–retest measure for stability?

4. Homogeneity is a measure of internal consistency. All items on the instrument should be complementary and should measure the same characteristics or concepts. Match each of the examples below with the appropriate test for homogeneity from the following list:

    1. Item-total correlations
    2. Split-half reliability
    3. Kuder-Richardson (KR-20) coefficient
    4. Cronbach's alpha

    a. _____ The odd items of the test had a high correlation with the even numbers of the test.

    b. _____ Each item on the test using a 5-point Likert scale had a moderate correlation with every other item on the test.

    c. _____ Each item on the test ranged in correlation with the total from 0.62 to 0.89.

    d. _____ Each item on the true–false test had a moderate correlation with every other item on the test.

5. Review the study by Babenko-Mould and Laschinger (2014) and answer the following questions:

   a. Think about the concept of reliability and about the variables addressed in the study. Comment on the reliability of the study tools. Was there any information given on the Chronbach's alpha to indicate the level of reliability?

   b. What information is given to the reader about the Maslach Burnout Inventory-General Survey (MBI-GS) (Schaufeli, Leiter, Maslach, et al., 1996)?

   c. Have the strengths and weaknesses of the reliability and validity of each instrument been presented?

Activity 4—Web-Based Activity

Click on the link https://www.cdc.gov/mmwr/preview/mmwrhtml/mm5108a3.htm to read an article by the Centers for Disease Control and Prevention: Health-Related Quality of Life—Puerto Rico, 1996–2000. Read the results and the limitations section of the article. What measures of rigour were used to validate the HRQOL?

Activity 5

Use the critiquing criteria listed in Chapter 14 of the textbook to think about the study by Laschinger (2014) described in Appendix B of the textbook. What methods were used to establish methodological rigour?

Activity 6

Use the critiquing criteria listed in Chapter 14 of the textbook to assess the study by Pauly, McCall, Browne, et al. (2015) described in Appendix C, and then answer the following questions:

1. How many instruments for data collection were used in this study?

2. What information on validity and reliability was provided for each instrument?

Activity 7—Evidence-Informed Practice Activity

Think about the study by Laschinger (2014) reviewed in Activity 5. Look at the study response rate. If you were a nurse from an acute care setting in a hospital in Ontario, how would you apply the study knowledge to guide your practice and decision making?

POST-TEST

Complete the sentences below with a term from the following list of types of validity and reliability. Terms may be used more than once.

content	test–retest
factor analysis	Cronbach's alpha
convergent	alternate- or parallel-form
divergent	interrater
concurrent	item-to-total correlation

1. In tests for reliability, the self-efficacy scale had a(n) _____ of 0.88, demonstrating internal consistency for the new measure.

2. The ABC social support scale demonstrated _____ validity with a correlation of 0.84 with the XYZ interpersonal relationships scale.

3. _____ validity was supported with a correlation of 0.42 between the ABC social support scale and the QRS loneliness scale.

4. The investigator established _____ validity through evaluation of the cardiac recovery scale by a panel of cardiac clinical nurse specialists. All items were rated from 0 to 5 for importance to recovery, and only items scoring above an average of 3 were kept in the final scale.

5. The results of the _____ were that all the items clustered around three factors, lending support to the notion that there are three dimensions of coping.

6. The observations were rated by three experts. The reliability among the observers was 94%.

7. To assess _____ reliability, subjects completed the locus-of-control questionnaire at the beginning of the project and 2 weeks later. The correlation of 0.86 supports the stability of the concept.

8. Bennett, Puntenney, Walker, et al. (1996) developed an instrument called the Cardiac Event Threat Questionnaire (CTQ). They (1) established _____ validity by reviewing the literature that described the concerns of patients recovering from a cardiac event, and (2) had the items critiqued by a panel of experts.

9. The results of the CTQ were highly correlated with the results of a test measuring negative emotions. This established _____ validity.

10. Bennett et al. (1996) reported that the internal consistency reliabilities of the five factors of the CTQ were computed with the _____ statistic.

11. In qualitative research, to what does the term *saturation* refer?
    a. Data repetition
    b. Subject exhaustion
    c. Researcher exhaustion
    d. Sample size

12. In qualitative research, data are often collected by which of the following procedures?
    a. Questionnaires sent to subjects
    b. Observation of subjects in natural settings
    c. Interviews
    d. All of the above

Please check with your instructor for the answers to the Post-Test.

REFERENCES

Babenko-Mould, Y., & Laschinger, H. (2014). Effects of incivility in clinical practice settings on nursing student burnout. *International Journal of Nursing Education Scholarship, 11*(1), 145–154. doi: 10.1515/ijnes-2014-0023

Bennett, S. J., Puntenney, P. J., Walker, N. L., et al. (1996). Development of an instrument to measure threat related to cardiac events. *Nursing Research, 45,* 266–270.

Cornelius, J., & Carrick, J. (2008). Survey of nursing students' knowledge and attitudes regarding LGBT health care concerns [Abstract]. Retrieved from https://stti.confex.com/stti/congrs08/tech-program/paper_38998.htm

Kelley, L., Chou, C. L., Dibble, S. L., et al. (2008). A critical intervention in lesbian, gay, bisexual, and transgender health: Knowledge and attitude outcomes among second-year medical students. *Teaching and Learning in Medicine: An International Journal, 20*(3), 248–253. doi: 10.1080/10401330802199567

Laschinger, H. K. S. (2014). Impact of workplace mistreatment on patient safety risk and nurse-assessed patient outcomes. *Journal of Nursing Administration, 44*(5), 284–290.

Liou, S-R., & Ching, C-Y. (2014). Developing and validating the Clinical Competence Questionnaire: A self-assessment instrument for upcoming baccalaureate nursing graduates. *Journal of Nursing Education and Practice, 4*(2). Retrieved from http://www.sciedu.ca/journal/index.php/jnep/article/view/2862/0

Pauly, B., McCall, J., Browne, A. J., et al. (2015). Toward cultural safety: Nurse and patient perceptions of illicit substance use in a hospitalized setting. *Advances in Nursing Science, 38*(2), 121–135.

Sanchez, N., Rabatin, J., Sanchez, J., et al. (2006). Medical students' ability to care for lesbian, gay, bisexual, and transgendered patients. *Family Medicine, 38*(1), 21–27.

Schaufeli, W. B., Leiter, M. P., Maslach, C., et al. (1996). Maslach Burnout Inventory general survey. In C. Maslach, S. E. Jackson, & M. P. Leiter (Eds.), The Maslach Burnout Inventory–test manual (3rd ed.) (pp. 22–26). Palo Alto, CA: Consulting Psychologists Press.

Sirisawasd, P., Chaiear, N., Johns, N. P., et al. (2014). Validation of the Thai version of a work-related quality of life scale in the nursing profession. *Safety and Health at Work, 5*(2), 80–85.

Wright, M., Creed, P., & Zimmer-Gembeck, M. (2010). The development and initial validation of a brief daily hassles scale suitable for use with adolescents. *European Journal of Psychological Assessment, 26*(3), 217–223.

Zhao, Y., Wong, C. K. H., Miu, H. Y. H., et al. (2016). Translation and validation of a condom self-efficacy scale (CSES) Chinese version. *AIDS Education and Prevention, 28*(6), 499–510.

15 Qualitative Data Analysis

INTRODUCTION

Qualitative data analysis is an iterative process. Unlike quantitative analysis, qualitative analysis does not have a prescribed canon, although many qualitative traditions have established processes and procedures for taking "raw" data and drawing meaning from them.

LEARNING OUTCOMES

On completion of this chapter, you will be able to do the following:
- Describe the processes of qualitative data analysis.
- Outline the steps common to qualitative data analysis.
- Describe how data are reduced to meaningful units (themes).
- Describe the process of identifying themes and categories and the relationships between them.
- Assess the validity of a data analysis from a study.

Activity 1

Match the terms in Column B with the appropriate definitions in Column A.

Column A	Column B
a. _____ Process of transforming the data from transcripts	1. Coding
b. _____ Grouping of data	2. Themes
c. _____ Process of recognizing emergent themes	3. Data reduction
d. _____ Computerized qualitative data management	4. Hyper research
e. _____ Marking of the text	5. Thematic analysis

Activity 2—Web-Based Activity

Go to the website at http://onlineqda.hud.ac.uk and read the text on the home page. From the menu at the top of the page, move the cursor to "Analysis." Click on "What is QDA?" in the drop-down menu. Read down to the section titled "What does qualitative analysis involve?" Click on "How and what to code." Read down to the section titled "Types of coding," and complete Interactive Exercises A and B.

Activity 3

Following is an extract from an interview conducted with a personal support worker (PSW) that explores the experience of caring for older persons living in long-term care facilities. For this study, the proposed research question was "What is the lived experience of caring for older persons with Alzheimer's disease and related disorders in a special care unit within a long-term care (LTC) facility from the perspective of personal support workers (PSW)"? The research methodology was descriptive phenomenology. The data-collection method involved semi-structured, face-to-face, in-depth interviews that were tape-recorded, took place in a private room within an LTC facility, were 30–90 minutes in length, and were conducted before or after a PSW's shift.

Review the transcript and use the table plus readings from Chapter 15 to complete the table. Please note that I = interview and RP = research participant.

I: I'm interested in learning about the experience of caring for older adults with Alzheimer's disease or related disorders in a long-term care facility.

RP: Mm hmm.

I: So the first question is very general. I'm wondering if we can just talk about what it's like to care for people with Alzheimer's and related disorders in a long-term care facility. If you can tell me what's it's like to be a PSW on a special care unit?

RP: Well, first you have to have good patience, you have to be very gentle, you have to be very quiet and you have to have good . . . good courage.

I: Good courage.

RP: Good courage. If you don't have good courage, sometimes things get in the way, but if you have good courage, everything is good for you.

I: That's an interesting word, *courage*.

RP: Yes, you have to have good courage. That is number one. Number two, you have to be very gentle, speak very quietly, and have good courage. You know, when you have good courage you do everything for these people, like, this lady is my mother. I have to take good care of her.

I: Okay.

RP: You know, so the work never feel hard. They never feel discouraged. You always have good energy to work.

I: Okay. Interesting. When I think of the word *courage*, I think of brave.

RP: Well, you call it, I say courage, good courage mean you have good energy, you have good strength, you're always happy to work.

I: Mm hmm.

RP: You have to have all these things in mind when you come to work. You focus on today is what I'm going to do for these people; so if you have the courage, you have the energy, your whole day is perfect.

I: And why is that so important on a special care unit?

RP: Because for me, I feel like I'm here to take good care of these people.

I: Mm hmm.

RP: And I find myself feeling happy working with them. So when you're happy working with them, you know, you have a hard task, sometime it's very hard, sometime you have to have good courage, so you go and do everything every day to suit your needs.

I: What makes it hard on those days?

RP: Sometimes it's very hard, especially when you come like sundowning in the evenings.

I: Mm hmm.

RP: They're very restless, very aggressive. So you have to train yourself to know how to deal with these people. You can't talk to them hard, very quietly. Rub their shoulder, rub their back, and make them feel like they're at home.

I: You train yourself.

A: Yes, to do all these things to help them.

I: Can you tell me more about that? How do you train yourself?

RP: Well, okay. I'm coming to work today. This is what I want to do for this resident that I'm taking care of. If I came here and they are aggressive, I give them a drink of water; I'll give them a glass of juice if I can get a glass of juice. Then I put them to sit. I rub their hair a little bit, I rub their shoulder and so that way they don't feel left out.

I: Mm hmm.

Table 1

Major Themes	Subthemes	Code

Compare your coding with a classmate's. Was your coding similar? Did all of the codes apply? Are there other codes you could have added?

Activity 4

Using a prepared list of questions, conduct a 15-minute interview with a friend or classmate about his or her experiences during the first week of nursing education. Record the interview, and transcribe it into text. Review the text, identify its themes, and create a coding scheme. Cut and condense the data into major and minor codes.

Activity 5

Select quotations from the text of the interview from Activity 4 to support the themes you identified in the data from that activity.

Activity 6

Develop a chart or diagram to display the relationships between your themes. Why did you choose one method over another?

Activity 7

Share your findings with the participant. Did your findings ring true? Did the participant find that your themes and model reflected his or her experiences?

POST-TEST

1. Refer to the studies by MacDonald, Martin-Misener, Steenbeek et al. (2015) and Pauley, McCall, Browne, et al. (2015), described in Appendices A and C, respectively, to answer the following questions:

   a. How did each study complete the data analysis?

   b. Did the authors use qualitative research software to assist with the analysis? If so, what software was used?

   c. How did the authors validate their interpretations and analysis of the data?

2. In the space after each statement in the following list, write *T* if the statement is true or *F* if the statement is false. Rewrite the false statements to make them true statements.

   a. Qualitative data analysis typically follows a series of prescribed steps. _____

   b. Qualitative data analysis always proceeds in a linear fashion. _____

   c. Qualitative research software is not limited to organizing data; it also provides preliminary analysis. _____

   d. Data reduction is the process of selecting, focusing, simplifying, abstracting, and transforming the data from field notes or transcriptions. _____

   e. Themes can be considered structured meaning units. _____

   f. Qualitative researchers tend to avoid using figures and charts to display data. _____

Please check with your instructor for the answers to the Post-Test.

REFERENCES

MacDonald, C., Martin-Misener, R., Steenbeek, A., et al. (2015). Honouring stories: Mi'kmaq women's experiences with Pap screening in Eastern Canada. *Canadian Journal of Nursing Research, 47*(1), 72–96.

Pauly, B., McCall, J., Browne, A. J., et al. (2015). Toward cultural safety: Nurse and patient perceptions of illicit substance use in a hospitalized setting. *Advances in Nursing Science, 38*(2), 121–135.

16 Quantitative Data Analysis

INTRODUCTION

Measurement is critical to any study. The practitioner is interested in the similarity between the measurements used in a study and those usually found in his or her practice. The researcher thinks about how to measure relevant variables while reading the literature and thinking through the theoretical rationale for the study. Both the practitioner and the researcher wonder how much faith they can put in the measurements reported.

Practitioners and researchers know that the perfect set of measurements does not exist. The researcher's task is to clearly define the variables, choose accurate measurement tools, and explain how the statistical tools were used. The task of a practitioner who reads research is to consider the researcher's explanation of how and why specific descriptive and inferential statistics were used and to ask, "What do these numbers tell me?"

Descriptive statistics are valuable for summarizing data and for assessing the salient features of a body of data, but practitioners usually want more information. They want to be able to read about an intervention used with a specific group of individuals and to consider the usefulness of that intervention for clients in their care. Inferential statistics provides a way for practitioners to look at the data in a study and decide how easily the results can be generalized to their everyday clients.

Initially, numbers tend to be intimidating. The best way to deal with this intimidation is to jump in and play with the numbers, reminding yourself that you have the intelligence and skills to do this. Also, remember that this is a lifelong learning process; there will still be times when you will read a study (e.g., one that adds a new twist to a statistical procedure) and have to go back to the reference books or consult a colleague.

This chapter is designed to help you with the skills part of the task. First, the exercises will give you some practice in working with the concept of measurement. Second, you will need to think through some decisions regarding descriptive and inferential statistics. Most of your effort will be spent digesting data from the studies included in the text.

LEARNING OUTCOMES

On completion of this chapter, you will be able to do the following:
- Differentiate between descriptive and inferential statistics.
- State the purposes of descriptive statistics.
- Identify the levels of measurement in a research study.
- Describe a frequency distribution.
- List measures of central tendency and their use.
- List measures of variability and their use.
- Identify the purpose of inferential statistics.
- Distinguish between a parameter and a statistic.
- Explain the concept of probability as it applies to the analysis of sample data.
- Distinguish between type I and type II errors and their effects on a study's outcome.
- Distinguish between parametric and nonparametric tests.
- List the commonly used statistical tests and their purposes.
- Critically analyze the statistics used in published research studies.

Activity 1

In this activity, you will create your own "statistical assistants" in the form of a set of reference cards that can also serve as flash cards. Once the cards are finished, carry them with you to the library, set them on the desk when you are on the Internet, or use them when reading research reports. Before long, you will be able to read a piece of research without referring to your statistical assistants, and you will have memorized the statistical notation. You will no longer have to flip through a book to find a statistical symbol before you can evaluate the use of a statistic.

Gather the following supplies: a package of 3 × 5-inch index cards lined on one side; six pens or a combination of pens and highlighters in six different colours; and one broad-tipped black ink marker.

1. Make two "key" cards first. On the unlined side of the first card, write "NAME OF INFERENTIAL STATISTICAL TECHNIQUE" with the black marker. Take the second card and write "NAME OF DESCRIPTIVE TECHNIQUE" on the unlined side.

2. Turn the first card (the one for inferential technique) over to the lined side. With one of the coloured pens, write "Symbol" on the first line. Complete this side of the card with five more categories of information, using a different line and a different-coloured pen for each line of each category, as in the following example:

Symbol	Parametric/nonparametric?
# of independent variables (IV)	# of dependent variables (DV)
IV's level of measurement	DV's level of measurement
HR = relationship? (# of variables?)	Differences? (# of groups?)

3. On the lined side of the second card, write the following:

   Symbol

   Central tendency

   Variability

   Frequency

   Each line of each key card should be a different colour.

4. Next, create a stack of "statistical assistants." On the unlined side of a card, write the full name of one statistical tool (for example, "Pearson product moment correlation") with the black marker.

5. Turn over the card, and write the information that corresponds to the appropriate category on the key card on the appropriate line with the appropriate coloured pen. If you need help with choosing the appropriate information to put on each line, refer to Table 16.1 and the Critical Thinking Decision Path in Chapter 16 of the text. For example, the lined side of the "Pearson product moment correlation" card would read as follows:

r

IV = 1

DV = 1

IV = at least interval

DV = at least interval

relationship (2 variables)

parametric

These cards will fit into an envelope or into small plastic cases that can be purchased from your local bookstore, and they can be slipped into a briefcase, backpack, or knapsack with ease.

Activity 2

Match the levels of measurement listed in Column B with the appropriate examples in Column A. Refer to Table 16.1 in the textbook for help, if necessary.

Column A

1. _____ Gender

2. _____ Scores on the ACT, Scholastic Aptitude Test (SAT), or Graduate Record Examination (GRE)

3. _____ Height or weight

4. _____ High, moderate, or low level of social support

5. _____ Satisfaction with nursing care

6. _____ Blood pressure

7. _____ Amount of empathy

8. _____ Number of feet or metres walked

9. _____ Blood types

10. _____ Body temperature measured with centigrade thermometer

Column B

a. Nominal

b. Ordinal

c. Interval

d. Ratio

Activity 3

If you have taken a course in statistics, you are familiar with the statistical notation used to refer to specific types of descriptive statistics. This activity will serve as a quick review. If you have not yet taken a statistics course, this exercise will provide you with the information needed to recognize some statistical notations.

The puzzle shown below is a *reverse* crossword puzzle; that is, the puzzle is already completed. Your task is to identify the appropriate clue (in the following list) for each word in the puzzle. In the list below the puzzle and clues, match the letter of each clue (e.g., a or d) to the number of its correct "across" or "down" square.

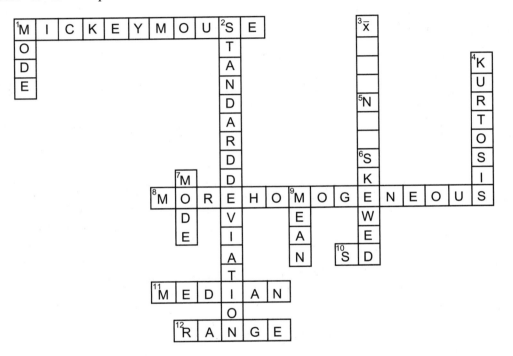

Clues

a. Measure of central tendency used with interval or ratio data
b. Abbreviation for the number of measures in a given data set (the measures may be individual people or some smaller pieces of data, such as blood pressure readings)
c. Measure of variation that shows the lowest and highest numbers in a data set
d. Can describe the height of a distribution
e. Old abbreviation for the mean
f. Marks the "score" where 50% of the scores are higher and 50% are lower
g. Describes a distribution characterized by a tail
h. Abbreviation for standard deviation
i. 68% of the values in a normal distribution fall within ± 1 of this statistic
j. Goofy's best friend

k. Very unstable

l. The values that occur most frequently in a data set

m. Describes a set of data with a standard deviation of 3 when compared with a set of data with a standard deviation of 12

Across	Down
1.	1.
3.	2.
5.	4.
8.	6.
10.	7.
11.	9.
12.	

Activity 4

Read the following excerpts from abstracts of specific studies. Identify both the independent and dependent variable(s), and indicate what level of measurement would apply. You may find the Critical Thinking Decision Path in the textbook helpful in completing this activity.

1. The purpose of this analysis was to determine correlates of exercise participation among adolescents. . . . A secondary analysis was conducted of data from a cross-sectional survey of 300 adolescents seen at an urban clinic. Using descriptive statistics and path analysis, we examined the direct and indirect effects of independent variables on exercise participation. (Ammouri, Kaur, Neuberger, et al., 2007)

   a. Name the variable of interest.

   b. Identify the level of measurement of this variable.

2. [The purpose of the study was] to evaluate quality of life (QOL) and cost outcomes of advanced practice nurses' (APNs') interventions with women diagnosed with breast cancer. . . . [W]e completed a randomized control trial. . . . The control group ($n = 104$) received standard medical care. The intervention group ($n = 106$) received standard care plus APN interventions. . . . QOL was measured using the Functional Assessment of Cancer Therapy, Mishel Uncertainty in Illness Scale, and Profile of Mood States at seven intervals over 2 years. Information about costs (charges and reimbursement) was collected through billing systems. (McCorkle, Dowd, Ercolano, et al., 2009)

   a. Name the independent variable(s).

   b. Name the dependent variable(s).

   c. Identify the level of measurement of each variable.

3. The aim of this prospective repeated measures, mixed-methods observational study was to assess whether depressive, anxiety, and stress symptoms are associated with postpartum relapse to smoking. . . . A total of 65 women who smoked prior to pregnancy and had not smoked during the last month of pregnancy were recruited at delivery and followed for 24 weeks. Surveys administered at baseline and at 2, 6, 12, and 24 weeks postpartum [were used to] assess smoking status and symptoms of depression (Beck Depression Inventory [BDI]), anxiety (Beck Anxiety Inventory [BAI]), and stress (Perceived Stress Scale [PSS]). (Park, Chang, Quinn, et al., 2009)

a. Name the independent variable(s).

b. Name the dependent variable(s).

Activity 5

Fill in the blank spaces in the statements below with the appropriate terms from the following list. Some terms may be used more than once.

ANOVA	correlation	logistic regression
null hypothesis	parameter	parametric statistics
practical significance	probability	measures of central tendency
sampling error	confidence interval	statistical significance
type I error	type II error	sample

1. The _____ states that there is no difference between the groups in the study or no association between the variables under study. It is useful to a study because it is the only relationship that can be tested with statistical tools.

2. _____ is an example of the use of _____.

3. _____ describe the characteristics of a sample.

4. The tendency for statistics to fluctuate from one sample to another is known as the _____.

5. The term _____ refers to a characteristic of the population, whereas the term _____ refers to a characteristic of a sample drawn from a population.

6. When investigators are studying the association between variables, they often use statistics that measure _____.

7. A _____ occurs when the investigator does not find a statistically significant difference but a real difference exists. A _____ occurs when the investigator concludes that there is a real (statistically significant) difference but in reality there is no difference.

8. The relative frequency of an event in repeated trials under similar conditions is known as _____ and provides the theoretical basis for inferential statistics.

9. A statistically significant finding of a change of 3 mm Hg in systolic blood pressure in a sample of healthy individuals would likely have little _____.

10. The relationships between independent variables and a dependent variable are tested through _____.

11. _____ is an estimated range of values, which is likely to include an unknown population parameter calculated from a given set of sample data.

12. When a probability level is $p < .05$ and the investigator has set the alpha level of significance at .05, the investigator must reject the _____ and accept the _____.

13. Identify the components of the following statistical test result:

$$\chi^2 \ (6, n = 213) = 33.0, p < .0001$$

Indicate the name of the component in the space before the component.

χ^2	a. Sample size
6	b. Degrees of freedom
$n = 213$	c. Chi-square symbol
33.0	d. Probability level
$p < .0001$	e. Chi-square test statistic

Activity 6

The table below contains data from a study. Use the statistical assistant cards you made in Activity 1 to answer the questions that follow the table.

Relationship of Postpartum Health to Demographic and Perinatal Variables

Variables	n	Postpartum Health* M + SD	Test	df	p-Value
This childbirth experience			$t = -3.38$	859	.01
Satisfying	784	2.09 ± 1.98			
Unsatisfying	77	2.89 ± 2.16			
Preferred sex of this baby			$t = 2.14$	660	.03
Had gender preference	345	2.35 ± 2.18			
No preference	516	2.04 ± 1.87			

Note: df = degrees of freedom; M = mean; SD = standard deviation.
From Hung, C. H. (2004). Predictors of postpartum women's health status. *Journal of Nursing Scholarship, 36*(4), 349.
*Scores on instrument used to measure postpartum health. Higher scores indicate poorer health status.

1. Explain what the researcher wants you to learn from the table.

2. What descriptive statistics are present in the table?

3. What inferential statistic was used with these data?

4. Name the independent variable(s) and the dependent variable(s).

5. What is the level of measurement for each of the variables named in question 4?

6. State the null hypothesis or hypotheses in this study.

Activity 7

Answer the following questions about the use of descriptive and inferential statistics in each of the studies described in Appendixes B and C in the textbook. Once again, use the Critical Thinking Decision Path in Chapter 16 of the textbook.

1. Were descriptive statistics used in these studies? (Answer for each study.)

    Laschinger (2014) (Appendix B) _____

    Pauly, McCall, Browne, et al. (2015) (Appendix C) _____

2. What data were summarized or explained through the use of descriptive statistics? (Answer for each study.)

    Appendix B _____

    Appendix C _____

3. Were the descriptive statistics used appropriately? (Answer for each study.)

    Appendix B _____

    Appendix C _____

4. Did one of the two studies rely more heavily on the use of descriptive statistics than the other? If so, why do you think this occurred?

5. In each study, was some type of inferential statistic used to manage the data?

    Appendix B _____

    Appendix C _____

6. Name the inferential statistical tools used in each study and the variables used with each inferential tool.

    Appendix B _____

    Appendix C _____

7. In which study was the data analysis easiest to read? Why was it easiest to read?

Activity 8—Web-Based Activity

Go to http://www.canadianwomen.org/facts-about-violence, and read the fact sheet on violence against women.

1. What percentage of women report spousal violence and sexual violence?

2. Compare the statistics of both women and men fearing for their lives in a context of spousal violence.

Activity 9—Evidence-Informed Practice Activity

Evidence-informed practice means basing practice decisions on the best evidence available. In an ideal world, practitioners would have available many experimental studies with clear conclusions that have direct relevance to an immediate clinical concern. Obviously, this is seldom the case. Practitioners must use their brains and the best practice information available to intervene and to evaluate.

Assume that the statistics from Activity 8 about violence against women have been consistently reported by several studies of varying designs and sample sizes. What implications (if any) would there be for nurses working in an emergency department?

POST-TEST

1. Two outpatient clinics measured client waiting time as one indicator of effectiveness. The mean and standard deviation of waiting time in minutes are reported below for each clinic.

	Clinic 1	Clinic 2
Mean (in minutes)	40	25
Standard deviation (in minutes)	10	45

Which outpatient clinic would you prefer, as a practitioner, assuming that all other things are equal? Explain your answer.

2. You are responsible for ordering a new supply of hospital gowns for your unit. Which measure of central tendency would be most useful in your decision making? Explain your answer.

3. Use the table below to answer the questions that follow. Each of the items was responded to as either true (scored as 1) or false (scored as 0).

Means and Standard Deviations on Survey Questions ($N = 116$)

	M	SD
Every Saturday night, a girl in your class has a party. She invites all your friends but never invites you. You are a victim of bullying.	.17	.38
One Friday, you wear a new dress to school, and your best friend tells you on the way to class that it makes you look fat. She is bullying you.	.67	.47
A girl in your class regularly starts rumours about people at school that are true. This girl is a bully.	.86	.35
A group of girls is passing notes in class, and when certain people raise their hands, all of the girls giggle. These girls are bullies.	.62	.49
When girls tease each other, it can have lasting effects on self-esteem and body image.	.95	.22
Bullies exist at my school.	.92	.27

Note: M = mean; SD = standard deviation.
From Raskauskas, J., & Stoltz, A. D. (2004). Identifying and intervening in relational aggression. *Journal of School Nursing, 20*(4), 211.

a. To which statement was there the widest range of responses? What statistic did you use to answer this question?

b. Which statements did the respondents (adolescent girls) agree with most? Explain your answer.

c. The incident described in the second item of the table was considered to be benign (i.e., not to be a bullying incident). How would you interpret the mean and the standard deviation associated with the responses to this item?

Please check with your instructor for the answers to the Post-Test.

REFERENCES

Ammouri, A. A., Kaur, H., Neuberger, G. B., et al. (2007). Correlates of exercise participation in adolescents. *Public Health Nursing, 24*(2), 111–120.

Laschinger, H. K. S. (2014). Impact of workplace mistreatment on patient safety risk and nurse-assessed patient outcomes. *Journal of Nursing Administration, 44*(5), 284–290.

McCorkle, R., Dowd, M., Ercolano, E., et al. (2009). Effects of a nursing intervention on quality of life outcomes in post-surgical women with gynecological cancers. *Psycho-Oncology, 18*(1), 62–70.

Park, E. R., Chang, Y., Quinn, V., et al. (2009). The association of depressive, anxiety, and stress symptoms and postpartum relapse to smoking: A longitudinal study. *Nicotine & Tobacco Research, 11*(6), 707.

Pauly, B., McCall, J., Browne, A. J., et al. (2015). Toward cultural safety: Nurse and patient perceptions of illicit substance use in a hospitalized setting. *Advances in Nursing Science, 38*(2), 121–135.

17 Presenting the Findings

INTRODUCTION

As the last sections of a research report, the Results and Conclusion sections answer the question, "So what?" In these two sections, the investigator "makes sense" of the research, critically synthesizes the data, ties the data to a theoretical framework, and builds on a body of knowledge. These sections are an important part of the research report because they describe the generalizability of the findings and offer recommendations for further research. Well-written, clear, and concise "Results" and "Conclusions" sections provide valuable information for nursing practice. Conversely, poorly written "Results" and "Conclusions" sections will leave a reader bewildered and confused and wondering how or if the findings are relevant to nursing.

LEARNING OUTCOMES

On completion of this chapter, you will be able to do the following:
- Discuss the difference between a study's "Results" section and the "Discussion" section.
- Identify the format of the "Results" section.
- Determine whether both statistically supported and statistically unsupported findings are discussed.
- Determine whether the results are objectively reported.
- Describe how tables and figures are used in a research report.
- List the criteria for a meaningful table.
- Identify the format and components of the "Discussion of the Results" section.
- Determine the purpose of the "Discussion" section.
- Discuss the importance of including the generalizations and limitations of a study in the report.
- Determine the purpose of including recommendations in the study report.
- Discuss how the strength, quality, and consistency of evidence provided by the findings are related to a study's limitations, generalizability, and applicability to practice.

Activity 1

Knowing what information to look for and where to find it in the "Results" and "Discussion" sections of a research report will enable you to interpret research findings and critique research reports.

Identify the section in which the following information in a research report may be found. Put an *R* in the blank space if the information would be found in the "Results" section and a *D* if the information would be found in the "Discussion" section.

1. _____ Tables and figures

2. _____ Limitations of the study

3. _____ Data analysis related to literature review

4. _____ Inferences or generalization of results

5. _____ Statistical support or nonsupport of hypotheses

6. _____ Findings of hypothesis testing

7. _____ Information about the statistical tests used to analyze hypotheses

8. _____ Application of meaning (i.e., making sense) of data analysis

9. _____ Suggestions for further research

10. _____ Recommendations for nursing practice

Activity 2

Tables are an important part of the data analysis component of a study. Review the following tables from the study by Hipolito, Samuels-Dennis, Shanmuganandapala, et al. (2014), which examined the protective functions of spirituality and personal empowerment in the relationship between childhood and adulthood experiences of violence and mental health/well-being among social assistance recipients in Ontario, Canada. Review the data in Tables 1 and 2 from the same study and answer the questions that follow the tables.

Of the 1,917 students, 71% were from Ontario and 29% were from Alberta. Age ranged from 13 to 16 years (mean = 14.72 [SD 0.72] years) (Table 1). Females were slightly overrepresented at 54%. Based on self-reported body mass index (BMI), 80%, 17%, and 3% of participants were classified as normal weight, overweight, and obese, respectively (Table 2). The prevalence of overweight and obesity was higher among male participants than among females ($\chi^2 = 59.9$ ($df = 2$), $p < 0.001$) (Vance, Woodruff, McCargar, et al., 2009).

Table 1. Demographic Frequencies and Percentages for the Full Sample and by Gender

Demographics	Total		Men		Women	
	n	*%*	*n*	*%*	*n*	*%*
Ethnicity						
Caucasian	64	20.3	26	23.0	38	18.8
Black	148	47.0	48	42.5	100	49.5
Asian	46	14.6	20	17.7	26	12.9
Hispanic	45	14.3	14	12.4	31	15.3
Multiracial/Other	12	3.8	5	4.4	7	3.5
Marital status						
Single/Never married	201	63.8	71	62.8	130	64.4
Married/Common law	48	15.2	23	20.4	25	12.4
Single (separated, divorced, widowed)	66	21.0	19	16.8	47	23.3
Level of education						
Grade school	11	3.5	6	5.3	5	2.5
High school	162	51.6	57	50.4	105	52.2
Post-secondary (partial)	36	11.5	10	8.8	26	12.9
Post-secondary	88	28.0	28	24.8	60	29.9
Some or completed graduate school	17	5.4	12	10.6	5	2.5

Note: From Hipolito, E., Samuels-Dennis, J. A., Shanmuganandapala, B., Maddoux, J., Paulson, R., Saugh, D., & Carnahan, B. (2014). Trauma-informed care: Accounting for the interconnected role of spirituality and empowerment in mental health promotion. *Journal of Spirituality in Mental Health,* *16*(3), 193–217.

Table 2. Frequencies and Percentages of Childhood Abuse and Intimate Partner Violence by Gender

Abuse Types	Men		Women	
	n	*%*	*n*	*%*
Childhood emotional abuse				
None	45	39.8	65	32.2
Low	23	20.4	34	16.8
Moderate	17	15.0	37	18.3
Severe	28	24.8	66	32.7
Childhood physical abuse				
None	51	45.1	85	42.1
Low	18	15.9	29	11.4
Moderate	14	12.4	26	12.9
Severe	30	26.5	68	33.7
Childhood sexual abuse				
None	81	71.7	98	48.5
Low	4	3.5	18	8.9
Moderate	15	13.3	25	12.4
Severe	13	11.5	61	30.2
Physical abuse				
No	52	46.0	68	33.7
Yes	61	54.0	134	66.3
Nonphysical abuse				
No	91	80.5	123	60.9
Yes	22	19.5	79	39.1

Note: From Hipolito, E., Samuels-Dennis, J. A., Shanmuganandapala, B., Maddoux, J., Paulson, R., Saugh, D., & Carnahan, B. (2014). Trauma-informed care: Accounting for the interconnected role of spirituality and empowerment in mental health promotion. *Journal of Spirituality in Mental Health, 16*(3), 193–217.

1. Does the information in the tables meet the criteria for a table as described in Chapter 17 of the textbook? Explain why it does or does not.

2. Conduct a simple Google Scholar search for general statistics on men's and women's exposure to violence. Is there a fair representation of violence exposure in the study? Explain your answer.

3. Which group was more likely to experience nonphysical violence?

4. Which group was more likely to experience childhood physical abuse?

Activity 3

Collect demographic data on the people in your research class. You can decide what data you want to collect, but common variables are age, gender, eye colour, hair colour (current or underlying), and so on. Once the data have been collected, work in groups of three to five members, and create a table that displays these data.

Exchange tables with another group, and critique each other's tables with the intent of improving them. Consider the following questions:

   a. Are data summaries included but not all of the raw data?
   b. Is the title clear? Without reading the text, can you tell what data are being presented?
   c. Are the columns and rows appropriately labelled?
   d. Are there other criteria you want to include? Does your instructor have suggestions?

Activity 4

1. Review Table 3 below from the article by Samuels-Dennis, Ford-Gilboe, and Ray (2011) and then answer the questions that follow.

Table 3. Sample Characteristics

Characteristics	Total Sample ($N = 247$)	
	n (%)	Mean (SD)
Age ($n = 245$)		35.7 (9.5)
Number of children ($n = 246$)		1.8 (1.04)
Marital status ($n = 244$)		
Single never married	137 (56.1)	
Separated/divorced	103 (42.2)	
Widowed	4 (1.6)	

Continued

Table 3. Sample Characteristics—cont'd

Characteristics	Total Sample (N = 247)	
	n (%)	**Mean (SD)**
Race/ethnicity (n = 234)		
Native/Aboriginal	12 (5.0)	
Black	63 (26.4)	
Caucasian	90 (37.7)	
East and Southeast Asian	10 (4.2)	
Pacific Islander/Filipino	1 (0.4)	
South Asian/East Indian	16 (6.7)	
Hispanic/Latin American	18 (7.5)	
Middle Eastern/Arab	6 (2.5)	
Biracial	18 (7.5)	
Education (n = 244)		
Less than high school	29 (11.9)	
High school graduate	95 (38.9)	
Some college/university	47 (19.3)	
College/university graduate	73 (29.9)	
Employment status (n = 246)		
Employed full time	15 (6.1)	
Employed part time	41 (16.7)	
Unemployed	190 (77.2)	
Immigration status (n = 247)		
Born in Canada	134 (54.3)	
Born outside Canada	113 (45.7)	

Note: From Samuels-Dennis, J. A., Ford-Gilboe, M., & Ray, S. (2011). Single mothers' adverse and traumatic experiences and post-traumatic stress symptoms. *Journal of Family Violence, 26*, 12.

a. What is the meaning of "137 (56.1%)" next to the "Single never married" category?

b. Is there a good representation of Native/Indigenous people?

c. After examining the distribution of people born in and outside Canada, would you be comfortable applying these findings to people living in a city like Toronto, Canada?

2. Review Table 4 below from the same article and answer the questions that follow:

Table 4. Zero Order Correlations, Means, and Standard Deviations, for Study Variables ($n = 171$)

	1	2	3	4	5	6	7
Adversity[a]	—						
Psychological[a]	.246**	—					
Assaultive[a]	.252**	.543**	—				
Intrusion/re-experiencing	.139*	.245**	.141*	—			
Avoidance/numbing	.128*	.434**	.277**	.633**	—		
Hyperarousal	.064	.332**	.246**	.538**	.710**	—	
Total PTSD	.129	.395**	.266**	.820**	.913**	.864**	—
Descriptive							
Mean	2.50	3.09	3.46	10.39	14.75	14.26	39.58
SD	1.89	2.13	2.53	10.82	13.52	13.52	31.44
Minimum, Maximum	0, 9	0, 9	0, 12	0, 40	0, 56	0, 56	0, 134

PTSD, post-traumatic stress disorder; SD, standard deviation.
[a]Lifetime exposure to multiple unique events.
*$p < .05$, **$p < .01$ (one-tailed).
Note: From Samuels-Dennis, J. A., Ford-Gilboe, M., & Ray, S. (2011). Single mothers' adverse and traumatic experiences and post-traumatic stress symptoms. *Journal of Family Violence, 26*, 15.

    a. What was the mean total PTSD score? What does it mean?

    b. Interpret the value ".710."

    c. How many variables are represented by the information provided in Table 4?

Activity 5—Web-Based Activity

1. Go to the website at http://www.google.com, and type "analysis" in the search box. Scroll down and look at the number of websites that use the word "analysis" in their titles. Look through a few pages (each page usually lists 10 sites). On a scale of 1 to 10 (with "1" indicating very little value), where would you place the value of using the word "analysis" as a search term when looking for studies relevant to nursing? Use various modifiers of "analysis" and see if you can get some useful information from this search.

2. Do a search after entering "analysis research studies, nursing" in the search box. How many site names appeared? Skim through the first five pages of listed sites. What words seem to be driving the search?

Activity 6—Evidence-Informed Practice Activity

Evidence-informed practice requires practitioners to use the best evidence available when deciding which interventions to use. The "Results" and "Discussion" sections of a study report can help practitioners decide whether the given study should be included in their considerations. Go to the website at http://hsl.lib.umn.edu/learn/ebp/ and click on "Lessons." Complete Lessons 1 and 2. What was the most significant new learning that occurred for you?

POST-TEST

1. When a research hypothesis is supported through testing, it may be assumed that it was which of the following?
   a. Proved
   b. Accepted
   c. Rejected
   d. Disconfirmed

2. The "limitations" of a study describe its weaknesses: true or false?

   True   False

3. The "Results" section of a research study includes all but which of the following?
   a. Results of hypothesis testing
   b. Tables and figures
   c. Descriptions of statistical tests
   d. Limitations of the study

4. "Unsupported hypotheses" means that the study is of little value in improving practice: true or false?

   True   False

5. Tables in research reports should meet all but which of the following criteria?
   a. Be clear and concise
   b. Restate the text
   c. "Economize" the text
   d. Supplement the text

6. The "Discussion" section of a research report provides the opportunity for the investigator to do all but which of the following?
   a. Describe the implications of the research results
   b. Relate the results to the literature review
   c. Generalize the research to larger populations
   d. Suggest areas for further research

7. Hypothesis testing is described in the "Discussion" section of a research report: true or false?

   True   False

Please check with your instructor for the answers to the Post-Test.

REFERENCES

Hipolito, E., Samuels-Dennis, J. A., Shanmuganandapala, B., et al. (2014). Trauma-informed care: Accounting for the interconnected role of spirituality and empowerment in mental heath promotion. *Journal of Spirituality in Mental Health, 6*(3), 193–217.

Samuels-Dennis, J. A., Ford-Gilboe, M., & Ray, S. (2011). Single mothers' adverse and traumatic experiences and post-traumatic stress symptoms. *Journal of Family Violence, 26,* 9–20.

Vance, V. A., Woodruff, S. J., McCargar, L. J., et al. (2009). Self-reported dietary energy intake of normal weight, overweight and obese adolescents. *Public Health Nutrition, 12*(02), 222–227.

18 Critiquing Qualitative Research

INTRODUCTION

Qualitative research can generate new knowledge about phenomena that are less easily studied with empirical or quantitative methods. Nurse researchers increasingly use qualitative methods to explore holistic phenomena that are less easily investigated with objective measures. In qualitative research, the data are less likely to involve numbers and will mostly include text derived from interviews, focus groups, observation, field notes, or other such sources. The data tend to be mostly narrative or written words that require content analysis rather than statistical analysis. The contributions of qualitative research to nursing knowledge make it important that nurses be able to evaluate and critique qualitative research reports.

This chapter describes the criteria for evaluating and critiquing qualitative research reports. Qualitative researchers should provide the "insider" (i.e., emic) view of the phenomenon being studied. They often use a more conversational tone than that found in quantitative research and use quotations to present the findings. Page limits in journals greatly constrain how investigators can present the richness of their data. Quotations must be exemplary in making themes understandable to the reader. Published research reports, whether quantitative or qualitative, must have scientific merit, demonstrate rigour in the research conducted, present new knowledge, and be of interest to the reader. Qualitative research should offer evidence to enhance understanding of or increase knowledge about a specific phenomenon; it may also have strong implications for the way in which nursing practice is thought about and delivered.

LEARNING OUTCOMES

On completion of this chapter, you will be able to do the following:
■ Identify the influence of stylistic considerations on the presentation of a qualitative research report.
■ Identify the criteria for critiquing a qualitative research report.
■ Evaluate the strengths and weaknesses of a qualitative research report.
■ Describe the applicability of the findings of a qualitative research report.
■ Construct a critique of a qualitative research report.

Activity 1

The methods of presentation in qualitative research reports are different from those in quantitative studies. Nurses writing qualitative research reports face the challenge of presenting the richness of the data while being bound by the restrictions of publication guidelines.

Review the articles in Appendices A and D in the textbook, and describe how the researchers presented the rich data. Carefully read the sections presenting the findings, and identify the descriptive examples or quotations that summarize the key points.

Activity 2

Critiquing qualitative research enables the nurse to make sense of the research report, build on the body of knowledge about human phenomena, and consider how that knowledge might be applicable to nursing. Learning and applying a critiquing process is the first part of this process.

1. Review Box 18.1 in the textbook, and then fill in the blank spaces next to the statements in Column B with the letters denoting the appropriate steps in Column A. Some steps are used more than once.

Column A

A. Participant selection

B. Study method

C. Researcher perspective

D. Data analysis

E. Application of findings

F. Description of findings

G. Study design

Column B

a. _____ The purpose of the study is clearly stated.

b. _____ Audio-recorded interviews are used to collect phenomenological data.

c. _____ The participants recognize the experience as their own.

d. _____ Purposive sampling is used.

e. _____ Data are clearly reported in the research report.

f. _____ The researcher has remained true to the findings.

g. _____ Recommendations for future research are made.

h. _____ The phenomenon of interest is clearly identified.

i. _____ Participant observation is done in an ethnography.

2. Define the following terms:

   a. Credibility

   b. Auditability

   c. Fittingness

   d. Saturation

   e. Trustworthiness

Activity 3—Web-Based Activity

The Internet can be a valuable tool for gaining insight into qualitative research topics. Searching with the term "qualitative research" can be a way to get a better understanding of this research approach. However, it is essential to identify a few quality starting points for your investigation.

The Association for Information Systems has a web page titled "Qualitative Research in Information Systems" (http://www.qual.auckland.ac.nz/) about the conduct, evaluation, and publication of qualitative research; this site contains valuable information about qualitative studies. The website of the University of Alberta's International Institute for Qualitative Methodology, at https://www.ualberta.ca/international-institute-for-qualitative-methodology, is an excellent site for getting information about conferences, journals, training, and international research. Another good site is "Qual Page" at https://qualpage.com/2016/08/01/qualpage-relaunched/, a valuable resource for learning more about the various methods of qualitative research. The Cochrane Collaboration (which maintains a website at http://www.cochrane.org/) is an international nonprofit organization whose purpose is to produce and disseminate reviews of health care interventions and clinical trials that provide evidence for practice. Spend some time reviewing these websites to learn more about qualitative research methods. Your instructor may assign specific activities from these sites to help you learn about qualitative research.

Activity 4

Complete each of the following sentences with the appropriate word or phrase from the text.

1. The full meaning or richness of the phenomenon being studied in qualitative studies is expressed by the inclusion of _____.

2. Identified themes are supported by quotes from the participants to establish _____.

3. When critiquing a study, the reviewer is examining the credibility, auditability, and _____ of the data.

4. The _____ view or insider's view of the phenomenon being studied is described in detail in most qualitative study reports.

5. Large quantities of data are often condensed into _____.

POST-TEST

For statements 1 through 6, indicate whether they are true (*T*) or false (*F*).

1. _____ Qualitative research findings are generalizable to other groups.

2. _____ Nurse researchers view findings from qualitative research designs as less credible than those from quantitative studies.

3. _____ Auditability is an important aspect of evaluating a qualitative research report.

4. _____ The style of a qualitative research report differs from that of a quantitative research report.

5. _____ Some journal publication guidelines may impede the qualitative researcher's ability to convey the richness of the data.

6. _____ Journal review guidelines usually allow for the extra pages that qualitative researchers might need to present their rich data in detail.

For statements 7 through 11, fill in the blank spaces with the appropriate word(s).

7. _____ is the important measure of rigour in qualitative research.

8. _____ means that others should be able to identify the thinking, decisions, and methods used by the researcher(s) when the study was conducted.

9. _____ means that the study findings are applicable outside of the study situation.

10. _____ is a term usually applied to qualitative research related to the validity and reliability of the data.

11. The four criteria proposed by Lincoln and Guba (1985) _____ formed the framework for determining the rigour of the research.

Please check with your instructor for the answers to the Post-Test.

REFERENCE

Lincoln, YS. & Guba, EG. (1985). Naturalistic Inquiry. Newbury Park, CA: Sage Publications.

19 Critiquing Quantitative Research

INTRODUCTION

Chapter 19 in the textbook includes two thorough critiques of quantitative studies. The authors address the various critiquing criteria presented in the previous chapters and carefully take the reader through each item. The result is a complete critique of two separate studies.

Both of these critiques reflect the level of analysis desired for an article relevant to nursing practice. To produce a critique with this degree of thoroughness takes time. It is not uncommon for a novice reader of research to take 2 to 3 hours (maybe longer) to complete writing such a critique. Usually, novice readers of research find the task tedious and difficult. The more often you read and critique studies in this manner, the easier (and more interesting) reading research becomes and the quicker it can be done.

One way to start mastering this skill is to work with a weekly schedule: each week, find one research article relevant to your favourite area of nursing, and critique that article by using the steps outlined in the textbook. At the end of one year, you will have read 52 studies and will have mastered the research critique.

As mentioned earlier, this level of reading and critiquing is most often used when there is a reasonable expectation that a specific study will be useful in professional practice. But not all relevant articles will be found in journals devoted specifically to your area of clinical interest. You must search several journals to find all of the articles that can be useful. When you do find an article that appears relevant to practice, assess the article quickly to decide whether it requires a more in-depth analysis.

LEARNING OUTCOMES

On completion of this chapter, you will be able to do the following:
- Identify the purpose of the critiquing process for a quantitative research report.
- Describe the criteria of each step of the critiquing process for a quantitative research report.
- Evaluate the strengths and weaknesses of a quantitative research report.
- Discuss the implications of the findings of a quantitative research report for nursing practice.
- Construct a critique of a quantitative research report.

Activity 1

The quick reading of study articles demands that one consider the same aspects of a study that one would consider in reading a more detailed critique, except in a more superficial manner. Adler and Van Doren (1972) called this type of reading "inspectional reading." Mastering inspectional reading is essential but is often overlooked as an analytical skill. Frequently, professional reading must be squeezed into a small window of available time. The ability to read quickly will help you sort through the reading material required to maintain and expand your knowledge.

But what is inspectional reading? It is the second level in a set of reading skills described by Adler and Van Doren (1972). Level one is elementary reading (usually learned by the time you have completed Grade 4). Level two is inspectional reading. Level three is analytical reading, in which the reader tries hard to understand what the author is attempting to share; this is the level of reading required to critique a research study. Level four is "syntopical" reading, which requires intense effort to synthesize ideas from many sources.

Inspectional reading has two components: systematic skimming and superficial reading.

Systematic skimming is the first thing to do when approaching a reading assignment. It requires only a few minutes to skim an article; it may take up to an hour to skim a complete book. To skim a research article in hard copy, you would do the following:

- Read the title and the abstract.
- Read the biographical information about the authors or researchers.
- Pay close attention to the clinical area and the population of subjects.
- Read the "Conclusions" section.
- Ask yourself, "Are the individuals in this study comparable to the people I am interested in? Is the problem, clinical area, or question close to my interests?" If you answer "no" to these questions, put down the study report and go on to the next one. If you answer "yes" to either of these questions or if you cannot decide whether the study is relevant to your clinical concerns, proceed to a superficial reading of the article.

Superficial reading requires that you read the article from beginning to end without stopping. Do not take notes. Do not highlight. Do not use the dictionary to look up words you do not know. Do not stop and think, "I wonder what they meant by that." Just read!

When you have finished reading the article, ask yourself the following questions:

1. Does it fit my interests?
2. What do I remember about the study? The question? The methods? The results? The discussion?
3. Was this clinical or basic research?
4. Was it experimental, nonexperimental, or qualitative?
5. How would I rate this study on the level-of-evidence scale?
6. Does the study raise any ethical questions? (If there is even a twinge of a question in this regard, pay attention to it.)

Generally, if the answer to the first question is "no," move on to the next article. If the answer is "maybe," put the article in a "come back to it later" stack. If the answer is "yes," then proceed to a more detailed reading and perhaps jot down notes that would be necessary to complete a critique or respond to questions 2 to 6.

Now for some practice. The article by Pauly, McCall, Browne, et al. (2015) in Appendix C of the textbook has been used for several activities in this study guide. If you have not read it from beginning to end, do so now, using the skills of inspectional reading. After reading the article, answer the questions that are related to superficial reading. Decide if this is an article that would help you build the evidence base for the area of nursing that most appeals to you.

When you have completed your reading, turn to the answers in the back of the Study Guide.

Note: There is no Post-Test for this chapter. Enjoy the break!

REFERENCES

Adler, M. J., & Van Doren, C. (1972). *How to read a book.* New York: Simon & Schuster.

Pauly, B., McCall, J., Browne, A. J., et al. (2015). Toward cultural safety: Nurse and patient perceptions of illicit substance use in a hospitalized setting. *Advances in Nursing Science, 38*(2), 121–135.

20 Developing an Evidence-Informed Practice

INTRODUCTION

Practitioners face two major obstacles in applying available evidence to practice. The first obstacle is finding the literature. The Internet has made this easier and more difficult at the same time. It is easier because instead of having to get to a library before it closes, one can simply turn on the computer and log on to the Internet. Internet searches can yield millions of articles, which is how the Internet has made searching for appropriate articles more difficult: There is simply too much to search. The second obstacle is thinking through the analytical strategies to determine the usefulness of a given study or group of studies. Both obstacles can be overcome. Help in searching the literature is available from the nearest health science librarian. Learning the analytical tools can be accomplished by thoroughly reading one study a month. Find a study in your clinical area of interest (the librarian can help). Use the analytical tools presented in Chapter 20 of the textbook, and work until you determine how much faith you can place in that particular study.

LEARNING OUTCOMES

On completion of this chapter, you will be able to do the following:

- Differentiate among conduct of nursing research, research utilization, and evidence-informed practice.
- Describe the steps of evidence-informed practice.
- Identify three barriers to evidence-informed practice and strategies to address each.
- List three sources for finding evidence.
- Describe strategies for implementing evidence-informed practice changes.
- Identify steps for evaluating an evidence-informed change in practice.
- Use research findings and other forms of evidence to improve the quality of care.

Activity 1

In each of the following scenarios, identify the relevant components of the mnemonic "PICOT" (patient, population, or problem; intervention/treatment; comparison intervention/treatment; outcome; time frame).

1. Janice is a nurse on a pediatric unit that encourages parents to spend nights in the hospital room with their ill child. She has noticed that fewer parents are staying overnight since the in-room recliners were replaced with convertible beds. Janice decides to develop a focused clinical question and, over the next 6 months, to ask all families to complete the questionnaire.

   P _____

   I _____

   C _____

   O _____

   T _____

2. Sam is a nurse on a hemodialysis unit. Patients are verbally instructed about diet and fluid restrictions, but 81% of the patients have trouble following the dietary restrictions, and 75% of them have difficulty following the fluid restrictions.

P _____

I _____

C _____

O _____

T _____

3. Sharon is a school nurse. Over the past 5 years, concern about overweight children has led the school board to consider eliminating vending machines that dispense snacks and soft drinks from the schools in the district.

P _____

I _____

C _____

O _____

T _____

Activity 2—Evidence-Informed Practice Activity

Several evidence-informed tools were discussed in Chapter 20 of the textbook. Specific concepts and techniques are associated with each tool. Write each term from the following list in the space beside the appropriate evidence-informed tool shown below the list. More than one term may fit a given tool.

librarian	PICOT	screening questions
therapy studies	diagnosis studies	information literacy
screening questions	meta-analysis	confidence intervals
Knowledge translation	likelihood ratios	evaluation

Tool 1: Asking a focused clinical question _____

_____

Tool 2: Searching the literature _____

_____

Tool 3: Synthesizing primary studies to form secondary knowledge _____

_____

Tool 4: Appraising each article's findings _____
_____

Tool 5: Applying knowledge to local context _____
_____

Activity 3—Web-Based Activity

Go to the website at http://www.cochrane.org. Review the links on this site to answer the following questions:

1. What are the Cochrane Reviews?

2. Why are the Cochrane Reviews useful to researchers and health care providers?

3. The free online abstracts can be very useful for informing practice. How can you search the abstracts?

4. How can you access the full text of reviews from The Cochrane Library? Which provinces or territories provide free access to the reviews?

5. Does your college or university provide you with access to The Cochrane Library systematic reviews?

POST-TEST

Mark each of the following statements as true (*T*) or false (*F*) in the blank space before each one. If a statement is false, rewrite it to make it a true statement.

1. _____ An experimental or quasiexperimental study design is usually used for the diagnosis category of clinical concern.

2. _____ Articles should be screened to determine if the setting and sample in the study are similar to those of your clinical situation.

3. _____ Dichotomous variables are also known as *outcomes*.

4. _____ A confidence interval can give the reader information about the statistical significance of the findings.

5. _____ *Specificity* describes the proportion of individuals with a disease who test positive for it.

6. _____ Odds ratio is a measure of association between an exposure and an outcome.

7. _____ Every study included in a meta-analysis is read by every member of an evidence-informed-practice team.

8. _____ Blobbogram is a new type of bubble gum.

9. _____ A meta-analysis synthesizes findings across many research studies.

Please check with your instructor for the answers to the Post-Test.

Answer Key

CHAPTER 1   THE ROLE OF RESEARCH IN NURSING

Activity 1
1. c
2. b
3. d
4. a
5. g
6. e
7. f

Activity 2
1. C
2. A, B, C
3. B, C
4. C
5. A
6. A
7. A
8. B
9. A, B

Activity 3

Activity 4—Evidence-Informed Practice Activity

Answers will vary.

Activity 5—Web-Based Activity

Answers will vary.

Activity 6

Following are possible answers.

1. In nursing, Carper's fundamental ways of knowing is a typology that attempts to classify the different sources from which knowledge and beliefs in professional practice can be or have been derived. *Empirical knowing* refers to factual knowledge from science, or other external sources, that can be empirically verified. Research aids in the development of a body of knowledge specific to nursing. Nursing research is important because it enables nurses to develop, test, and validate theories relevant to nursing practice. Research supports health promotion activities and specifies the type of care that might be most helpful in specific settings (i.e., acute versus community). It is also important because it aids in the development of valid interventions for multiple dimensions of illness and health.

2. Answers will vary.

3. Answers will vary with the topic of interest. Articles relevant to the types of knowledge that inform nursing practice would be helpful. Research that speaks to the causes of specific illness and test interventions would make for good conversations. If, for instance, your area of practice is psychiatric/mental health nursing with an emphasis on chemical dependency, you would want to have research findings demonstrating that nursing interventions related to "increasing knowledge about addiction" have an effect on the outcome of increased sobriety for the addict or alcoholic.

CHAPTER 2 THEORETICAL FRAMEWORK

Activity 1

a. Epistemology: A branch of philosophy that deals with what we know as truth or knowledge and includes its origins, limits, and nature.

b. Ontology: A branch of philosophy that studies the nature of being or existence.

c. Concept: A set of abstract ideas representing the fundamental characteristics of phenomena.

d. Theoretical framework: A structure that can hold or support a theory of a research study that explains why a phenomenon (that thing of interest) under study exists.

e. Paradigm: From the Greek word meaning "pattern," it has come to describe how a person or a group of people thinks about the world.

f. Constructivism: The basis for naturalistic (qualitative) research that is guided by the ontological perspective and suggests that many realities exist rather than only a single reality.

g. Post-positivism: Truth is sought through replicable observations, based on the premise that a single reality exists.

Activity 2

a. Theoretical knowledge: Theoretical knowledge is concerned with the developing or testing of theories or ideas that nurse researchers have about how the world operates.

Example: An example from your text (Chapter 2) is the study by Erci et al. (2003), who hypothesized that nursing care guided by Jean Watson's theory of human caring would improve patient outcomes such as quality of life (QOL) and blood pressure (BP).

Empirical knowledge: Empirical knowing involves observations and measurements of reality.

Example: Erci et al. (2003) developed an experiment that allowed them to observe BP measured every 3 months among patients who did and did not receive care guided by Watson's theory.

b. Quantitative research: The quantitative approach to research is based on the belief that we can best understand humans and their behaviour by taking the human apart. We study specific characteristics one at a time. We measure each one as we go, in the hopes that we can understand each characteristic in a clear and context-free manner. Once we clearly understand all of the pieces, we can put them together and understand the whole. Authors of quantitative studies rely much more heavily on preselected instruments, collect lots of data, and answer questions through the analysis of numbers that represent those characteristics.

c. Qualitative research: The qualitative approach to research is an accepted way of discovering knowledge that uses naturalistic investigation to learn about human phenomena. This method of research is grounded in the social sciences and provides nurses with ways to better understand the lived experience and human processes that surround health and illness.

Activity 3

Here is an example of how a researcher might view the problem of pain management differently based on whether he or she assumed a constructivist or post-positivist perspective.

If pain management associated with cancer is considered using a post-positivist paradigm, the approach might be to measure the physiological nature of pain mechanisms or the efficacy of a specific drug protocol versus an alternative therapy. In this case, it is highly likely that the researcher would select a research design with several groups, including a control group. The purpose would be to investigate the effects of various treatments on pain relief. The researcher may identify a large number of study participants using participant eligibility based on gender, race, ethnicity, and age in order to identify whether these variables make a difference in pain relief.

Research question: Are alternative pain management strategies such as touch therapy more effective than traditional strategies such as pharmacotherapy in helping patients manage their pain after surgery?

However, if one chooses to use a constructivist approach to investigate the problem, then the number of participants would likely be far smaller and might even be more homogenous in nature. For example, the investigator may want to describe the experience of pain management in Black women. The purpose of the study might be to explain the realities of living with cancer pain in women who are using alternative therapies.

Research question: What is the daily experience of living with pain among Black women suffering with cancer?

Activity 4

1. a. Inductive thinking moves from the particular to the general (or conclusions are developed from specific observations).

   b. Deductive thinking moves from the general to the particular (or predictions are developed from known relationships).

2. a. Inductive
   b. Deductive

3. Observations will vary. If you were able to write a general statement about "headache pain," you used inductive thinking and probably wrote something like:

   X (grimacing) X (rubbing temples) X (grumpy) = indications of headache pain.

   If you were unable to write a general statement, it could be that you do not know anyone who has headaches, so you don't have a database.

Activity 5—Evidence-Informed Practice Activity

1. a. Medication administration, web course, efficacy, nursing students, self-evaluate competence

   b. Undergraduate nurses/midwives, perceptions, spirituality/spiritual care, perceived competence

   c. Nursing students, Swedish, burnout, nursing program, upper year, 1 year post-graduation

   d. Disadvantaged youth, difficult situations, automatic responses

   e. Effectiveness, low-cost, smoking, intervention, pregnant women, brief counselling, prenatal care providers, self-help booklet, resource-intensive, cognitive-behavioural program

2. a. *Health promotion* is a concept. *Nursing diagnosis* is a construct.

   b. *Health promotion* and *nursing diagnosis* are similar in that both describe an abstraction. Both terms describe some notion that people want to be able to discuss, think about, or use without spending hours describing what is meant.

   c. The terms are different in one important dimension. *Health promotion* is a concept that all people recognize, although the precise characteristics of health promotion may vary from person to person. The construct *nursing diagnosis* is an abstraction that has been created by a specific discipline to explain a concept that is unique to that discipline. Researchers in all disciplines, especially researchers within a given discipline, create constructs to structure their world of study.

3. Answers will vary. An argument could be made for the following as constructs: illness uncertainty, social support intervention, and verbal abuse.

4. Answers will vary.

Activity 6

B. Concept #1: *Workplace bullying* refers to "repeated and prolonged exposure to predominantly psychological mistreatment, directed at a target who is typically teased, badgered, and insulted, and who perceives himself or herself as not having the opportunity to retaliate 'in kind'" (Hauge et al., 2009, p. 350). Operational definition: Bullying was measured by the Negative Acts Questionnaire Revised (NAQ-R), which taps perceived exposure to three types of bullying at work (work-related, personal, and physical intimidation) (Einarsen & Hoel, 2001). The NAQ consists of 22 items rated on a 5-point Likert scale ranging from 1 = never to 5 = daily.

Concept #2: *Workplace incivility* refers to low-intensity rude or disrespectful behaviours with an ambiguous intent to harm others (Anderson et al., 1999). Operational definition: Cortina's Workplace Incivility Scale (Cortina, Magley, Williams, et al., 2001) was modified to create three scales based on specific sources of uncivil behaviour: supervisor, coworker, and physician. Seven items were assessed in reference to the frequency of exposure to uncivil behaviours from each source of incivility in the past 6 months using a scale ranging from 1 = never to 5 = daily.

Concept #3: *Job performance* refers to the quality of patient care provided. Operational definition: Perceived quality of patient care

outcomes was evaluated through three dimensions: (1) patient safety risk—assessed to tap nurses' perceptions of the effects of negative interpersonal interactions in the work unit related to patient safety using a 5-point Likert scale, i.e., rate on the extent to which they agreed with statements such as "negative interpersonal relationships on my unit create a risk to patient safety," "result in failure to report errors in patient care," and "threaten communication about patient care within the healthcare team"; (2) nurse-assessed adverse events—the scale developed by Sochalski (2001) was used, which consists of five items to assess nurses' perceptions of the frequency of common adverse patient outcomes over the past year (medication errors, nosocomial infections, falls, work-related injury, and patient complaints) on a scale from 1 = never to 4 = frequently; (3) perception of patient care quality—Aiken et al.'s (1994) Magnet hospital study was used to evaluate the quality of care of their respective unit on a scale ranging from 1 (poor) to 4 (excellent).

C. Concept #1 *Illicit substance use* refers to the use of drugs that are currently considered illegal in the Canadian context, such as marijuana, heroin, cocaine/crack, and methamphetamine. There are no clear operational definitions.

Concept #2 *Culturally safe care* is an approach to care that requires health care providers at all levels of organizations to (1) reflect on their own, often unconsciously held, attitudes and beliefs about others; (2) examine the ways in which history, social relations, and politics continue to shape people's responses, needs, access, and health; and (3) demonstrate flexibility in how they relate with others, especially those that differ from themselves. There are no clear operational definitions.

Activity 7

1. a. 4
   b. 5
   c. 6
   d. 4
   e. 1 or 3
   f. 1 or 3

g. 6
h. 1
i. 2
2. a. Deductive
b. Yes
c. None of the above

CHAPTER 3 CRITICAL READING STRATEGIES: OVERVIEW OF THE RESEARCH PROCESS

Activity 1
1. rational
2. active; inner
3. the point of view of the writer
4. nursing
5. three (or four)

Activity 2
1. b
2. b
3. a
4. b
5. a
6. a

Activity 3
1. a. Preliminary understanding
   b. Comprehensive understanding
   c. Analysis understanding
   d. Synthesis understanding
2. a. Read the article for the fourth time.
   b. Review your notes on the copy.
   c. Summarize the study in your own words.
   d. Complete one handwritten 12.5−20 cm card per study.
   e. Staple the summary to the top of the copied article.

Activity 4
1. C: Yes; D: No
2. C: Yes; D: No
3. C: Yes; D: No
4. C: Yes; D: No
5. C: Yes; D: No
6. C: Yes; D: No
7. C: Yes; D: No
   Summary C: I would categorize this study as quantitative—RCT

Summary D: I would categorize this study as qualitative—Ethnographic study

Activity 5—Web-Based Activity
a. Answers for this activity will vary.
b. Answers for this activity will vary.
c. Answers for this activity will vary.
d. Answers for this activity will vary.

Activity 6—Evidence-Informed Practice Activity
1. 8
2. 4 or 5 [this quote attends to both study design and sample size]
3. 8 [report findings generally include a discussion section relevant to plans for future studies]
4. 2
5. 7

CHAPTER 4 DEVELOPING RESEARCH QUESTIONS, HYPOTHESES, AND CLINICAL QUESTIONS

Activity 1
1. e
2. d
3. b
4. d
5. a
6. c

Activity 2
Study A: a. Yes; b. No; c. Yes; d. Yes
Study B: a. Yes; b. Yes; c. Yes; d. Yes
Study C: a. Yes; b. No; c. No; d. Yes

Activity 3
1. a. CRTs
   b. Birth defects
2. a. Birth defects
   b. Independence–dependence conflicts
3. a. White wine
   b. Serum cholesterol level
4. a. Type of recording
   b. Patient care
5. a. Profession (physician or nurse)
   b. Extended-role concept for nurses

Activity 4

1. Hr, DH
2. Hr, DH
3. RQ
4. Hr, DH
5. Hr, NDH

Activity 5

1. RQ: Does the use of CRTs by pregnant women influence the incidence of birth defects?
   Ho: The use of CRTs by pregnant women has no effect on the incidence of birth defects.
2. DH: Individuals with birth defects have a higher incidence of independence–dependence conflicts than individuals without birth defects.
   NDH: There is a difference in the number of independence–dependence conflicts between individuals with and without birth defects.
   Hr: As is.
   RQ: Do individuals with birth defects have a higher incidence of independence–dependence conflicts than those without birth defects?
   Ho: There is no difference in the incidence of independence–dependence conflicts between individuals with and without birth defects.
3. DH: There is a positive relationship between daily moderate consumption of white wine and serum cholesterol levels.
   NDH: Daily moderate consumption of white wine influences serum cholesterol levels.
   Hr: There is a relationship between daily moderate consumption of white wine and serum cholesterol levels.
   RQ: As is.
   Ho: There is no relationship between daily moderate consumption of white wine and serum cholesterol levels.

Activity 6

1. a. Yes
   b. Yes
   c. Yes
   d. Yes
   e. Yes
   f. Yes
2. a. Yes
   b. Yes
   c. Yes
   d. Yes
   e. Yes
   f. Yes
   g. Yes

Activity 7—Evidence-Informed Practice Activity

Yes. The significance would be related to the relationship between the cost of patient care technicians (PCTs) and nurses (PCTs are less costly), and patient outcomes in terms of satisfaction, morbidity, and mortality. Remember that one would need to assume that a thorough literature review did not provide an answer.

Activity 8

The research question poses the question the researcher is asking. The hypothesis attempts to answer the question posed by the research problem. The research question does not predict a relationship between two or more variables.

CHAPTER 5   FINDING AND APPRAISING THE LITERATURE

Activity 1

1. research
2. education
3. research; practice
4. theory

Activity 2

1. c
2. a, b, d, f
3. e, f
4. d
5. e
6. b, e

Activity 3

Any of the following scholarly nursing journals may be listed:
Advances in Nursing Science
Applied Nursing Research
Canadian Journal of Nursing Research
Canadian Journal on Aging
Canadian Journal of Neuroscience Nursing (formerly AXON)
Canadian Journal of Nursing Leadership
Canadian Journal of Public Health

Canadian Nurse
Canadian Oncology Nursing Journal
Canadian Operating Room Journal
Clinical Nurse Specialist
Clinical Nursing Research
Evidence Based Nursing
Geriatric Nursing
International Journal of Nursing Studies
Issues in Comprehensive Pediatric Nursing
Issues in Mental Health Nursing
Journal of Advanced Nursing
Journal of Clinical Nursing
Journal of Neonatal Nursing
Journal of Nursing Administration (JONA)
Journal of Nursing Care Quality
Journal of Nursing Education
Journal of Nursing Scholarship (formerly Image: Journal of Nursing Scholarship)
Journal of Obstetric, Gynecologic and Neonatal Nursing
Journal of Professional Nursing
Journal of Qualitative Research
Journal of Transcultural Nursing
Nurse Educator
Nursing Management
Nursing Outlook
Nursing Research
Nursing Science Quarterly
Qualitative Health Research
Research in Nursing & Health
Scholarly Inquiry for Nursing Practice
Western Journal of Nursing Research

Activity 4

1. C, No Title offered; D, Background
2. 1. C, Yes; D, Yes
   2. C, inadequate search strategy details; D, inadequate search strategy details
   3. C, ethnographic methodology not specifically outlined; D, Yes—lactation model
   4. C, Yes; D, Yes
   5. C, inadequately developed; D, Yes
   6. C, No; D, Yes
   7. C, No; D, Yes
   8. C, Yes; D, Yes
   9. C, Yes; D, purpose comes after literature review
   10. C, Yes; D, No

a. Summary of Strengths and Limitations for Pauly et al. (2015): Strong introduction that ends with the research question and the goal of the study. The review begins with an identified social-problem justification for the study: "A growing body of evidence shows that people who use illicit drugs, particularly when this intersects with visible markers of poverty . . . experience high rates of discrimination, stigmatization, and social exclusion in the health care sector." The issue of power and stigma is problematized and connected to the central concept of cultural safety. Limitations include the repetition of information, limited research versus theoretical literature, and limited overview of what is known and unknown in this field of study.

b. Summary of Strengths and Limitations for Héon et al. (2016): Strong introduction that clearly outlines the problem at hand. Extensive review of both theoretical and empirical literature. Focus on what is known, unknown, and research gaps. Offers critical appraisal of current literature and builds a case for the current study. Nice overview of theoretical framework.

3. Nineteen of 52 articles were less than 5 years old at the time this article was published. The literature review, like that in most qualitative studies, does not rely heavily on empirical literature (i.e., primarily conceptual literature is presented). This helps to control the influence of prior research on data analysis and the interpretation of findings. The flow of the story is hampered by repetition and a focus on definitions rather than being an exploration of what is known and unknown. The authors clearly establish a need for the study.

Activity 5

1. a. S
   b. P
   c. S
   d. S
   e. P
   f. P
   g. P

2. False
3. False
4. True
5. b; MEDLINE does not contain all nursing references like CINAHL does
6. True
7. True

Activity 6

1. Primary
2. Primary
3. Secondary

Activity 7

1. What is the source of the material?
   (*Note:* Look at the last term in the URL address to find the organizational name (it is often three letters long); possibilities include *.com* for a commercial organization, *.edu* for an educational institution, *.gov* for a government body*, .int* for an international organization, *.mil* for U.S. military, *.net* for a networking organization, *.ca* for Canada, and *.org* for anything else (usually a non-profit organization). Information gathered from an *.edu* or *.gov* source is most reliable.
2. Is the source a well-respected medical or nursing institution or a federal agency, or is the source an individual putting out his or her own opinion? Critique the source.
3. Is the researcher(s) name and his or her degree listed?
4. Is there a mechanism given to obtain further information about the study or the information presented?
5. Is enough data given in the web publication to make a critical analysis about the material? (*Note*: Remember, in a refereed, professional journal, usually three independent nursing experts in the field have reviewed the article in a blind review process to determine that this material merits publication.)

Activity 9—Evidence-Informed Practice Activity

Answers will vary. Review possible responses with your instructor.

CHAPTER 6   LEGAL AND ETHICAL ISSUES

Activity 1

1. Nursing research committee
2. Informed consent
3. Anonymity
4. Research ethics board
5. Justice
6. Unethical research study

Activity 2

1. Beneficence
2. Justice
3. Respect for person

Activity 3

Elements of Informed Consent
  1. Title of protocol √
  2. Invitation to participate √
  3. Basis for participant selection 0
  4. Overall purpose of the study √
  5. Explanation of benefits √
  6. Description of risks and discomforts √
  7. Potential benefits √
  8. Alternatives to participation √
  9. Financial obligations √
  10. Assurance of confidentiality √
  11. Compensation in case of injury 0
  12. Participant withdrawal √
  13. Offer to answer questions √
  14. Concluding consent statement 0
  15. Identification of investigators √

Activity 4

1. Older adults
2. Children
3. Pregnant women
4. The unborn
Other correct responses include those who are emotionally or physically disabled, prisoners, the deceased, students, and people with AIDS.

Activity 5

1. a, c, d, f, g
2. a, b, c, d, f, g (Also, presume "e" was not adhered to because the study began in 1932 before REBs and formal consent were required.)

Activity 6—Evidence-Informed Practice Activity

1. Appendix A: MacDonald, Martin-Misener, Steenbeek, et al. (2015): Ethical approval was obtained from the University Health Sciences Human Research Ethics Committee at Dalhousie University, Mi'kmaq Ethics Watch at Cape Breton University, and Mi'kmaq community leaders. The OCAP (ownership, control, access, and procession) principles (1998) and the Canadian Institutes of Health Research (2007) guidelines for health research involving Indigenous people were also followed.

2. Appendix B: Laschinger (2014): Ethical approval was obtained from Health Sciences Human Research Ethics Board at Western University.

3. Appendix C: Pauly, McCall, Browne, et al. (2015): The study obtained ethical approval from the University of Victoria and the University of British Columbia, as well as from the hospital site where the study was conducted. Informed consent was obtained from all participants prior to both in-depth interviews and participant observation.

4. Appendix D: Héon, Goulet, Garofalo, et al. (2016): Ethical approval was obtained from the research ethics board at Sainte-Justine University Hospital Center.

CHAPTER 7 INTRODUCTION TO QUALITATIVE RESEARCH

Activity 1—Web-Based Activity

1. a. Grounded theory: A research method that enables the investigator to discover a theory from systematically obtained data. The data come from the observations of the participants being studied. The purpose of this research is to generate a theory.

   b. Case study: A research method that provides an in-depth description of the phenomena of interest to the investigator. Data for case studies may come from a variety of sources. This research method provides a way to study complex phenomena that are poorly understood.

   c. Phenomenological research: A research method that examines naturalistic experiences as they are lived and understood as reality by human beings. Researchers examine phenomena that are of special interest to nursing. The goal of this research method is to understand experience from the perspective of those having the experience.

   d. Ethnographic research: A research method initially developed by anthropologists to study the ways human beings react within a cultural setting or experience it. The goal of this research method is to combine the emic (insider) with the etic (outsider) perspective. Nurses have used an adaptation called *ethnomethod* to study health and illness within a variety of cultural contexts.

2. (Your answers may not be identical, but may include similar ideas.)

   a. Grounded theory: This research method is useful for nurses as they search for knowledge about social behaviours. Methods often used in this type of research are unstructured interviews or conversation with a purpose. Data are analyzed using abstract categories until saturation is reached or no new information is being discovered.

   b. Case study: This research method uses in-depth interviews with participants and key informants, medical record reviews, observation, and excerpts from personal diaries or writings. In a way, case studies are life histories that enable the investigator to gain knowledge as he or she studies a person or phenomenon of concern over a long period of time. Case study designs must have five components: (a) the research question(s), (b) its propositions, (c) its unit(s) of analysis, (d) a determination of how data are linked to the propositions, and (e) criteria to interpret the findings.

   c. Phenomenological research: Phenomenology entails listening and truly hearing what people are saying in order to understand the lived experience from the perspective of the other. This type of research requires an attitude of inquiry that includes radical openness and extreme attentiveness to the world we live in. In order to do this type of research, the investigator must bracket or put aside his or her experience.

d. Ethnographic research: The goal of ethnographic research is to look for patterns, themes, connections, and relationships that have meanings for the people involved. Questions of interest in the ethnographic process are "What is this?" "What is happening in this subculture?" In order to gain access and complete an ethnographic study, the researcher usually identifies key informants or "insiders" who can provide access to others who can help tell the story.

Activity 2

1. f
2. e
3. a
4. b
5. b
6. d
7. c

Activity 3

1. naturalistic
2. Text
3. social processes
4. interviews and observations
5. explanatory
6. Historical
7. Leininger

Activity 4

Appendix A: Qualitative, participatory action research
Appendix B: Quantitative, cross-sectional study
Appendix C: Qualitative, ethnographic design
Appendix D: Quantitative, quasiexperimental

Activity 5—Evidence-Informed Practice Activity

1. Grounded theory
2. The goal of grounded theory is to generate a theory that describes or accounts for a pattern of behaviour (i.e. a social process) that is relevant and problematic to nursing and other disciplines.

Activity 6—Web-Based Activity

(In order to complete this activity, you must read the essay entitled "How Can We Argue for Evidence in Nursing?" at http://www.contemporarynurse.com/archives/vol/11/issue/1/ article/1496/how-can-we-argue-for-evidence-in-nursing.)

Consider what kinds of evidence you might need to adequately care for all the needs of a young woman with type 1 diabetes who has suffered the complications of blindness and kidney failure and spends 3 days a week associating with very ill elderly individuals on dialysis. Although much of her care may be related to the hemodialysis and physiological responses of her body to this medical procedure, nurses are also concerned about the holistic needs of patients. What kinds of evidence do you think might be needed to enable a nurse to provide optimal or excellent care for this patient? What kinds of evidence might you need to know about caregivers, the family household, adjusting to blindness, socialization needs, and other aspects of abilities to accomplish activities of daily living? What kinds of contributions might researchers using qualitative methods make to identify the kinds of interventions needed? The evidence that nurses need to provide optimal nursing care for the whole person may not be fully provided through quantitative studies. Qualitative research that explores the behavioural, emotional, and spiritual aspects of living with illness is needed, so that we can truly identify what might be the best nursing approaches for meeting specific care needs. This is an area where nurses will make large contributions in the next few decades.

CHAPTER 8 QUALITATIVE APPROACHES TO RESEARCH

Activity 1

1. a. scientific; artistic
   b. natural settings
   c. day-to-day life
   d. lived experience
   e. less
   f. everyday living; human uniqueness
   g. research question
   h. fit

2. a. B
   b. A
   c. D
   d. G
   e. C
   f. I
   g. J
   h. E
   i. H
   j. F
3. a. Element 1: Identifying the phenomenon
   1. Phenomenology: Study of day-to-day existence for a particular group of people.
   2. Grounded theory: Interested in social processes from the perspective of human interactions.
   3. Ethnography: Study of the complex cultural aspects related to a phenomenon.
   4. Historical research: An approach for understanding a past event.
   5. Case study: A focus on an individual, a family, a community, an organization, or some other complex phenomenon.
   6. Participatory action research: A systematic study or assessment of a community to plan context-appropriate action.
   b. Element 2: Structuring the study
   1. Phenomenology: Query is the lived experience, research perspective is bracketed, sample has either lived or is living the experience being investigated.
   2. Grounded theory: Questions address basic social processes and tend to be action oriented; researcher brings some knowledge of the literature but exhaustive review is not done before beginning the research. The researcher has concerns about contextual values, and the data are the essence of the theory that emerges. The sample would be participants who have had experience with the circumstances, events, or incidents being studied.
   3. Ethnography: Questions are about "lifeways," or patterns of behaviour, within a social or cultural context. The researcher attempts to make sense of the world from an insider's point of view. The researcher becomes the interpreter of events and tries to understand things from an emic point of view. Researchers do this by making their own beliefs explicit and setting aside their own biases or assumptions in order to better understand a different world view. The sample often consists of key informants who have knowledge, status, and the communication skills needed to describe the phenomenon being studied.
   4. Historical research: Questions are implicit and embedded in the phenomenon studied; the researcher understands the information without imposing interpretation. It is important for the researcher to clearly and carefully identify the event(s) being studied. Data used for the study may be of a primary or secondary nature.
   5. Case study: Questions about issues that serve as a foundation to uncover complexity and pursue understanding. The perspective of the researcher is reflected in the questions. Researchers may choose the most common cases or instead select the most unusual ones.
   6. Participatory action research: Questions in this form of research are framed around the ideas of "look." Look has to do with identification of the stakeholders and understanding the problems from their perspective.
   c. Element 3: Gathering the data
   1. Phenomenology: Written or oral data may be collected.
   2. Grounded theory: Collect data through audio-recorded and transcribed interviews and skilled observations
   3. Ethnography: Participant observation, immersion, informant interviews
   4. Historical research: Use of primary and secondary data sources
   5. Case study: Use of interviews, observations, document reviews, and other methods

6. Participatory action research: Seeks to engage stakeholders in discovering the answers to the community problems
  d. Element 4: Analyzing the data
  1. Phenomenology: Move from the participant's description to the researcher's synthesis
  2. Grounded theory: Data collection and analysis occur simultaneously and use theoretical sampling, constant comparative method, and axial coding.
  3. Ethnography: Data are collected and analyzed simultaneously, searching for symbolic categories.
  4. Historical research: Analyze for importance and then validity (authenticity) and reliability.
  5. Case study: Reflecting and revising meanings.
  6. Participatory action research: This stage of research is the "think" phase and is where what has been learned is interpreted or analyzed. The research has the role of linking the ideas provided by the stakeholders in an understandable way so that evidence for specific ways to address the problem can be provided to the community group.
  e. Element 5: Describing the findings
  1. Phenomenology: A narrative elaboration of the lived experience.
  2. Grounded theory: Descriptive language to show theory connections to the data.
  3. Ethnography: Large quantities of data; researchers provide examples from the data and propositions about relationships of phenomena.
  4. Historical research: Well-synthesized chronicle.
  5. Case study: Chronologically developed cases, a story that describes case dimensions or vignettes that emphasize various aspects of the case.
  6. Participatory action research: Information obtained in earlier research stages sets the stage for community planning, implementation, and evaluation.

Activity 2
Answers will vary.

Activity 3
  a. D
  b. C
  c. B
  d. A
  e. B
  f. E
  g. C
  h. D
  i. A
  j. C
  k. E
  l. C
  m. D
  n. C
  o. B
  p. A
  q. E
  r. A (could also be true of B or C)
  s. C
  t. C (could also be true of A)
  u. B

Activity 4—Evidence-Informed Practice Activity
Responses will vary. Discuss your responses with your course instructor.

Activity 5—Web-Based Activity
  a. An important feature of grounded theory is theoretical sensitivity, which refers to a personal quality of the researcher and relates to understanding the meaning and subtlety of data. Theoretical sensitivity has been described by Glaser and Strauss (1967) as the process of developing the insight with which a researcher comes to the research situation. By gaining theoretical sensitivity, the researcher will be able to recognize important data and formulate conceptually dense theory.
  b. Grounded theory is a research method developed by Glaser and Strauss (1967). It is a research approach used to develop a theory about a social process. The theory is developed after using a systematic approach to viewing and interpreting qualitative data

(observations, interviews). The theory is developed and evolves during the research process through the interplay between data collection and analysis phases (remember the iterative process). It is important to remember that the result of a grounded theory study is the generation of a *theory*, which incorporates a set of proposed beliefs about the relationships between concepts (themes) identified during the research process.

c. Unlike other qualitative methods, grounded theory uses both an inductive and a deductive approach.

CHAPTER 9   INTRODUCTION TO QUANTITATIVE RESEARCH

Activity 1

1. h
2. j
3. e
4. g
5. d
6. f
7. b
8. a
9. c

Activity 2

1. Instrumentation: The use of a standardized self-evaluation tool as opposed to one recently developed by the researcher would increase the internal validity of the findings. History: The addition of the web course as well as the new online self-evaluation tool are occurring together and may limit the interpretation of the findings. Use of a control group and randomization would improve interpretation of the findings.

2. Selection bias: Convenience sample even across countries can bias the study findings. Groupings of study according to perceived levels of spiritual care competence are needed to strengthen this design.

3. Testing: Taking the test repeatedly may be the factor leading to an increase in confidence and accuracy, rather than the experimental program. The use of different outcome instruments and measures may be necessary.

4. Mortality: The lack of full participation suggests that some people became engaged in the program while others did not. The high mortality rate suggests many things: the demands of the intervention may be too high; accessibility may be an issue; cultural safety and competence issues may be involved. It is important to look at the makeup of the final study sample when the results are interpreted.

5. Maturation: As women move through their pregnancy they might be less inclined to smoke. It would be good to examine the findings among groups of women at various stages of pregnancy. Of central concern is the fact that everyone in the study received some type of intervention. A control group that received no intervention at all would strengthen the findings of the study.

Activity 3

a. The setting consisted of a 65-bed neonatal intensive care unit in a university teaching hospital in Montreal, Canada.

b. The participants were 40 breastfeeding mothers (ages ≥18 years) of very or extremely preterm infants (p. 533).

c. The sample was selected using convenience sampling. The principal investigator approached eligible mothers within 24 hours after birth, explained the study, and obtained their informed written consent (p. 533). After obtaining consent, the mothers were randomly assigned to the intervention or control group (p. 534).

d. All necessary information was provided, including the inclusion and exclusion criteria, the process for acquiring consent, and a detailed explanation of the intervention.

e. The groups were homogenous. Review of table 1 (p. 539) reveals no significant differences across the control and intervention group relevant to ethnicity, education level, annual income, partnership, breastfeeding experience, or the timing of decisions about breastfeeding.

f. The variables were measured using self-report (i.e., diary of frequency and duration of breastfeeding), instruments that assessed breast milk quantity and quality. Constancy of measurement was supported training mothers, keeping breast milk frozen, and using lab assays (p. 535).

g. Twenty mothers served as the control group and received standard care, while 20 mothers served as the intervention group and received breast milk expression education and support intervention.

Activity 4

a. Is the design appropriate?
The authors offer the following as their statement of purpose: "The aim of this study was to investigate the impact of subtle forms of workplace mistreatment (bullying and incivility) on Canadian nurses' perceptions of patient safety risk and, ultimately, nurse-assessed quality and prevalence of adverse events" (p. 284). Impact may be assessed using numerous study designs, including correlational design, pre- and post-facto design, and experimental designs. For the specified aim and study setting, it is appropriate to use a correlational or cross-sectional design. The authors do not actually specify the design type.

b. Is the control consistent with the research design?
Control measures were consistent with the design. This was not an experiment, so the most important way to apply control was to ensure that the instruments used were valid and reliable. Obtaining a homogenous sample would be one additional method of control.

c. Think about the feasibility of this study. Is this a study that would be expected of a master's student in nursing? Of a doctoral student? Explain the reasoning behind your answer.
Feasibility speaks to time, money, expertise, access to participants, facilities and equipment, and ethics. This study uses data from a larger study of nurses working in acute care hospitals across Ontario in the fall of 2012. The study might be expected of a doctoral student, but not a master's student. The time required for the study, the Ontario-wide scope, the need to access a population that is not readily accessible, and the level of expertise required would be at the doctoral level at least. But more than likely this study would be completed by a well-established nurse scientist.

d. Does the design logically flow from the problem, framework, literature review, and hypothesis?
Yes. The author clearly outlines the problem: "Recently, scholars have identified the detrimental effects of seemingly minor forms of workplace violence, such as incivility or bulling" (p. 284) . . . and . . . "A growing body of knowledge in the management field has linked bullying and workplace incivility to numerous negative work outcomes, including increased turnover intentions, poor mental health, and absenteeism" (p. 285). The author next presents literature that helps us to understand the extent of the problem, what we know, what we do not know, and how this study might add to the field of study. The study is guided by Einarsen and Mikkelsen's model of workplace bullying, which is used to develop and test the hypotheses. The study design logically flows from the each of the aforementioned elements.

e. What were the threats to internal validity, and how did the investigators control for each?
Correlational studies are especially susceptible to threats to internal validity. There is no real way to overcome this other than changing the design. However, the current design was adequate for addressing the research question.

f. What were the threats to external validity, and how did the investigators control for each?
Selection bias is a major threat to external validity. The researchers attempted to overcome this challenge by ensuring that the sample was randomly selected by the College of Nurses of Ontario. Random selection attempts to ensure that the selected participants of the study resemble the population to which they would generalize their findings.

Activity 5—Evidence-Informed Practice Activity

1. Level I: *(C)* quantitative
2. Level II: *(C)* quantitative
3. Level III: *(C)* quantitative
4. Level IV: *(C)* quantitative

5. Level V: *(B)* qualitative, *(C)* quantitative, *(D)* a combination of qualitative and quantitative
6. Level VI: *(B)* qualitative, *(C)* quantitative, *(D)* a combination of qualitative and quantitative, or *(E)* anecdotal.
7. Level VII: *(A)* expert opinion, *(E)* anecdotal

Activity 6—Web-Based Activity

a. The purpose of the study was to provide an overall picture or description of single mothers' exposure to various types of stressful, adverse, or traumatic events and to look at how the mothers' current symptoms of PTSD relate to exposure in childhood and adulthood.
b. This was a community sample.
c. The participants were single mothers who were active recipients of social assistance.
d. The sample was randomly selected from a list of current recipients.
e. There was no treatment, as this was not an intervention.
f. Random selection was used as a measure of control.

CHAPTER 10   EXPERIMENTAL AND QUASIEXPERIMENTAL DESIGNS

Activity 1

1. Experimental
2. Solomon four-group
3. Time series
4. After-only experiment
5. After-only nonequivalent control group
6. True experiment
7. Nonequivalent control group

Activity 2

2. The nurses would be randomly assigned to each of the groups using a table of random numbers or computer random assignment.
3. The pain knowledge and attitudes questionnaire would be used as a pretest.
4. The teaching program is the experimental treatment.
5. The pain knowledge and attitudes questionnaire is also the post-test or outcome measure.
6. The Solomon four-group design is ideal for experimental studies in which the pretest might affect the outcome. In this case, the questionnaire might change nurses' knowledge and attitudes about pain management. The researcher will be able to compare results for nurses receiving the teaching and those not receiving the teaching, with and without the pretest.
7. This type of design is particularly effective in ruling out threats to internal validity that the before-and-after groups may experience. It is effective for highly sensitive issues that might be affected by simply completing a questionnaire as a baseline pretest.
8. A disadvantage of the Solomon four-group design is that a large number of participants must be available for assignment into the four groups.

Activity 3

1. a. Repeated measures or time series design, one group
   b. To quote the investigators, "the time series design is an effective research technique for evaluating social programs for the elderly when a separate control group is not feasible. Unwillingness to randomly assign persons seeking adult day programs

1.

	Pretest	Teaching	Post-Test
Group A	__X__	__X__	__X__
Group B	_____	__X__	__X__
Group C	__X__	_____	__X__
Group D	_____	_____	__X__

Note: The groups may be arranged in any order, but the four-group pattern must be followed.

to receive service or not, and the logistical and cost requirements of identifying and following a non-random group of those not seeking services, prohibited the use of a separate control group" (Warren, Ross-Kerr, Smith, & Godkin, 2003, p. 213).

2. a. Time series design
   b. This type of design is useful in determining trends. Data are collected for a baseline, the experimental treatment is introduced, and data are collected multiple times afterward to determine a change from baseline. In longitudinal studies, each participant can be compared with him- or herself over time so that trends can be observed. In this study, follow-up data were collected only twice. If there had been more data collection points, alternative explanations for the results, such as history effects, could have been ruled out.
   c. The disadvantages of this quasiexperimental design are that threats of selection and maturation cannot be ruled out. There is also a testing threat to validity due to multiple data-collection points.

Activity 4

1. a. Experimental designs are the most appropriate design for testing cause-and-effect relationships because the design enables the researcher to control the experimental situation. Therefore, experimental designs offer better corroboration than if the independent variable is manipulated in such a way that certain consequences can be expected. Such studies are important because one of nursing's major research priorities is documenting outcomes to provide a basis for changing or supporting current nursing practice. However, experimental designs are not commonly used in nursing research, for practical reasons.
   b. Quasiexperimental designs are usually more practical, more feasible, and more adaptable to real-world practice. In many studies important to nursing, for practical or ethical reasons it is not possible to randomize participants into groups.

2. The researcher must carefully examine other factors that could account for differences between groups.
3. The clinician must carefully critique the research study and look for other factors that might explain the results of the study. The results of any study with any design must be evaluated to determine if other factors influence the findings. The results should also be compared with the findings of similar studies.

Activity 5—Web-Based Activity

1. This number will vary depending on when the search is conducted.
2. This is not an actual study but a review article. The authors state that "the purpose of the presentation is to identify various approaches to the design of control groups in experimental studies."
3. This number will vary depending on when the search is conducted.
4. a. This is a randomized controlled trial with a prospective experimental design. The study was carried out in Tehran, Islamic Republic of Iran, between 2006 and 2007.
   b. A block randomization strategy was used in the study. Eligible women were randomized into two groups. Groups of women in different categories of age and education level were randomly assigned to intervention or control groups separately.
   c. The authors highlight one study limitation. The study was not sufficiently diverse to make generalizations to other women because of the characteristics of the study sample.
   d. The characteristics of the study sample (e.g., highly educated, predominantly unemployed, healthy married women intending to become pregnant within 1 year) may limit the generalizability to other women. The authors suggest that this type of intervention be replicated in a more diverse sample.

Activity 6—Evidence-Informed Practice Activity

1. Level IV
2. Level VI

CHAPTER 11   NONEXPERIMENTAL DESIGNS

Activity 1

```
L  O  N  G  I  T  U  D  I  N  A  L  D  M  E
C  I  S  P  U  E  Q  W  H  X  O  I  Y  H  X
C  R  F  L  G  Y  Q  E  R  C  X  E  C  G  P
U  W  O  L  Z  S  B  Q  F  H  V  O  H  H  O
N  T  L  S  C  I  S  Z  A  R  R  O  I  U  S
L  G  T  R  S  D  L  D  U  R  Z  L  D  O  T
U  E  I  O  I  S  Q  S  E  D  L  V  W  O  F
I  U  W  S  J  J  E  L  O  S  Y  U  H  I  A
G  T  D  K  X  O  A  C  I  E  M  D  I  I  C
Q  W  R  E  E  T  O  K  T  T  E  S  T  A  T
A  S  A  M  I  K  E  N  B  I  B  H  U  L  O
D  U  O  O  K  L  H  N  P  H  O  B  Z  V  F
M  C  N  G  U  L  U  E  O  L  Y  N  R  K  C
K  A  M  F  G  U  P  Q  S  B  Z  L  A  H  T
L  W  J  F  V  N  E  W  J  S  W  L  E  L  V
```

1. Survey
2. Longitudinal
3. Correlational
4. Ex post facto
5. Cross-sectional
6. Correlational
7. Longitudinal
8. Survey
9. Cross-sectional
10. Cross-sectional

Activity 2

	Advantages	Disadvantages
Correlational	A3	D1, D3, D4, D7
Cross-sectional	A1, A7	D2, D5, D6
Ex post facto	A4	D1, D2, D3, D4, D5, D7
Longitudinal	A2, A5	D2, D8, D9
Prospective	A2, A6	D3, D4, D7, D8
Retrospective	A4	D1, D2, D3, D4, D5, D7
Survey	A1	D5, D7

Activity 3

1. Prospective
2. Cross-sectional/survey comparative
3. Longitudinal or prospective
4. Survey comparative
5. Meta-analysis

Activity 4

1. Design: descriptive, exploratory
2. Yes, one of the major points of the text was that consumers must be wary of nonexperimental studies that make causal claims about the findings unless a causal modelling technique is used, which was not used in the Mohr study. It appears that the author may have attempted to state that a cause-and-effect relationship among the variables exists, which is not appropriate for an exploratory, nonexperimental study.

Activity 5

Ex post facto design

Activity 6—Web-Based Activity

1. Answers for this activity will vary depending on when the search is conducted.
2. Answers for this activity will vary depending on when the search is conducted.
3. Answers for this activity will vary depending on when the search is conducted.

Activity 7—Evidence-Informed Practice Activity

1. d
2. b
3. a, b

CHAPTER 12   SAMPLING

Activity 1

1. N
2. N
3. P
4. N
5. P
6. P
7. P

Activity 2

1. b
2. f
3. d
4. a
5. c
6. d
7. e
8. d

Activity 3

1. a. Yes
   b. Yes
   c. Random selection
   d. Probability sampling
   e. Yes
2. The advantage is that it ensures that everyone has an equal chance of being included in the study.
3. Even with random selection, the sample may not always represent the population to which the researcher wants to generalize the finding.
4. If the sample is representative for all senior nurse leaders, then the finding reported by the authors is a true reflection of what is happening in the clinical setting. The implication provided by the authors can be used to improve the clinical environment and the senior nurse leader's decision-making process.

Activity 4

1. True
2. True
3. False
4. False
5. True
6. True
7. False

Activity 5

1. Yes, the characteristics of the sample were well described.
2. Yes, the parameters of the population for this study would be patients experiencing major depressive symptoms or PTSD.

3. The study uses self-referring population, so it's not representative.
4. The criteria are very specific, and exclusion criteria are identified.
5. Yes, the study purposively excludes individuals who have severe mental health problems, such as schizophrenia or suicidal ideations.
6. It may be possible to replicate the study sample if there were a similar population available in the proposed study geographic areas.
7. The target population is the residents in a selected community in Ontario. The method was appropriate for the randomized control trial.
8. No bias is identified in the study.
9. The sample size is appropriate. The study provides justification for sample size calculation. The estimated number of participants required and the minimum number of participants needed are given.
10. Yes, approval was obtained from the research ethics board of each institution.
11. Yes, they defined the limitations of the study—especially, they did not selectively recruit residents who have a severe stress profile, and they discussed the impacts of this selection on the generalization of the study findings. They also took the participation of some other concurrent community campaign into consideration. Its influence on the study outcomes was highlighted.
12. The study mentions at the end that a knowledge translation plan was created. Study findings and key learnings will be communicated to community leader partners to ensure the transferring of the project to all of Ontario and potentially to all of Canada.

Activity 6—Web-Based Activity

The sample and sampling strategy is one variable that will influence the strength of the evidence provided by the study. The evidence from a meta-analysis of all *randomized* controlled trials is more influential in making practice change decisions than that from a single descriptive or qualitative study with a convenience sample.

CHAPTER 13   DATA COLLECTION METHODS

Activity 1

Study 1: MacDonald, Martin-Misener, Steenbeek, et al. (2015). (Appendix A)
1. c
2. It gave an in-depth understanding of the issue at hand and the contextual factors that influence life and health.
3.

Study 2: Laschinger (2014) (Appendix B)
1. d
2. It allowed for very quick collection of large amounts of data.
3. The response rate was low and could compromise external validity of the findings.

Study 3: Pauly, McCall, Browne, et al. (2015) (Appendix C)
1. b
2. Observations went beyond personal stories and impressions and allowed the researchers to articulate their observations while authentically attending to the environmental context that influences people's behaviour. Methods allowed the researchers to comprehensively address the research question.

Study 4: Héon, Goulet, Garofalo, et al. (2016) (Appendix D)
1. a, b, d, e
2. Mothers kept a diary of the frequency and duration of their breast milk expression. This self-observation method allowed for privacy and reduced costs compared to those for outsider observations. Lab assays were used to objectively assess the quality of mother's milk. Medical records and a written questionnaire were used to capture demographic and confounding variable data.
3.

Activity 2

```
D E L I V E R S T A T I S T C S Y E S P A S
S S A C A B I N E T F O R K A Z O S P E I O
I A W O P E R A T I O N A L I Z A T I O N B
G T S N O R N E V E R B Y D N E A U X B T J
N S Y S T E M A T I C A J H T B S D V S E E
I F L I K E R T S C A L E E R R O Y A E R C
F A K S C A L E S N O V N O C A A U L R R T
H C U T A C R A T I M A P V E T P U I V A I
Y T B E B H I R T E M A H V W K I C D A T V
P C O N T E N T A N A L Y S I S P V O T E I
R O Y C B K D S I S R T S A D V A N E I R T
E R E Y O D U G K A T P I B I O I O G O R Y
A V S I B R Q U E S T I O N N A I R E N E C
C I A R E S E A R C H L L R E A C E S O L O
T O B M E X C E L A E O O D A T A C O V I N
I U E A E V A L I D S T G N O S T O O E A S
V N Y E S S I N T E R V I E W S A R F R B U
I H A P P I E N E S S P C A T A G D U N I M
T X C I T E D E L P H I A T O T P S N V L E
Y C E A T U B B S A N D L D O N N M A R I R
Y A B L E A C O N C E A L M E N T O O T T S
A I K E V A L I K E I I A B C O N S U M Y S
```

1. Consumers
2. Physiological
3. Reactivity
4. Interviews
5. Records
6. Questionnaire
7. Objectivity, consistency
8. Concealment
9. Interrater reliability
10. Operationalization
11. Likert scale
12. Content analysis
13. Fun

Activity 3

1. Children; interactions between people where the investigator is not part of the interaction; psychiatric patients; classroom students
2. The consent is usually of the type where permission to observe for a specified purpose is requested. The specific behaviours to be observed are not named. The use of the data and degree of anonymity are explained. In some situations, the participants will be asked to review the data after the observation and before inclusion in the data pool.
3. Reactivity is the major concern, when the investigator has reason to believe that his or her presence will change the nature of the participants' behaviour.

Activity 4

Physiological measures would be of minimal use since the data being sought would not involve actual measures of the residents' physiological status. A researcher would not be particularly interested in current blood pressure, temperature, urinary output, etc.

One could consider using observation, for example, sitting in an emergency room and observing the types of health care concerns that people bring there. One would need to think about whether this would be observation with concealment and would need to wrestle with the notion of what is private information and what is public domain information.

The researcher could use questionnaires and collect data from all types of health care providers, which could result in a lot of data being provided in a short time. How busy would they be and what would be the probability of their filling out the questionnaire?

One could use an interview. It is costly in terms of researcher time but could provide more detailed information because participants could be asked to expand on specific items. But who should be interviewed? How does one get into their offices and homes?

The researcher would need to get some information from the people who actually live here. How could a cross-section of those individuals be reached? Could they be called? What about those people without a telephone?

It would be good to check out the census data to get a clearer picture of what is being dealt with. Probably there would be some morbidity and mortality data collected by the public health departments. Existing records could be used to get a first sense of what the parameters of "health" are in this community. Then find out who knows the most about this area and arrange some interviews with these individuals. These would be guided interviews with open-ended items to encourage the sharing of as much information as possible. One would also seek a way to collect data from a variety of health care users, for example, surveys in the waiting room of various agencies, maybe the crowd at a mall or at a community fair.

One data collection instrument would not be sufficient to collect the information needed about the areas addressed.

Activity 5
1. d
2. a
3. d
4. a, b, c
5. d

CHAPTER 14   RIGOUR IN RESEARCH

Activity 1
1. S; avoid error by proper calibration of the scale.
2. S; decrease error by providing instructions, ensuring confidentiality, or other means to allow students to freely express themselves.
3. R; lessen error by training research assistants and using strict protocols or rule books to guide analysis.
4. R; decrease their anxiety by addressing their concerns, providing comfort measures, or using other efforts that might decrease their anxiety. Anxiety may alter the test responses.

Activity 2
1. Construct validity; construct validity
2. Face validity
3. Content validity
4. Hypothesis-testing, and/or convergent and divergent, and/or contrasted-groups, and/or factor-analytical (Any three)
5. Construct validity and convergent validity
6. Construct validity
7. Content validity

Activity 3
1. Stability; homogeneity; equivalence
2. Test–retest methods could be accomplished by giving the same test again at a later date and seeing if the two scores are highly correlated. Parallel or alternative forms, such as alternative versions of the same test, could also be used to establish stability.
3. Alternative forms would be better if the test-taker is likely to remember and be influenced by the items or the answers from the first test.
4. a. 2
   b. 4
   c. 1
   d. 3
5. a. Reliability of the Cortina Incivility Scale (CIS) tool has been tested in Smith et al. (2010)'s study and indicated Chronbach's alpha reliability $\alpha = .85 - .89$. The authors indicated that reliability of the Emotional Exhaustion (EE) and Cynicism (C) subscales of the Maslach Burnout Inventory-General

Survey (MBI-GS) has been tested in numerous studies, but information about Chronbach's alpha was not offered.

b. The authors used Emotional Exhaustion (EE) and Cynicism (C) subscales to assess nursing student burnout. A 7-point Likert scale was used to measure this variable. Information regarding reliability and validity was provided.

c. The study does not offer enough information on the strengths and weaknesses of the reliability and validity of each instrument in the study.

Activity 4—Web-Based Activity

For reliability, internal consistency and test–retest (stability) were done. Content, construct, and concurrent validity were established.

Activity 5

Methods used to establish methodological rigour were selection of the entire population of the hospital that met the study criteria, followed by random selection of senior nurse leaders within units and use of established instruments.

Activity 6

1. The study used in-depth interviews with a purposive sample of nurses and patients, participant observation, and the reviewing of hospital policy documents to collect data.

The Transcript:

I: I'm interested in learning about the experience of caring for elderly people with Alzheimer's disease or related disorders in a long-term care facility.

RP: Mm hmm. } Primary question

I: So the first question is very general. I'm wondering if we can just talk about what it's like to care for people with Alzheimer's and related disorders in a long-term care facility. If you can tell me what's it's like to be a PSW on a special care unit? } Paraphrased question . . . might have muddied the water.

RP: Well, first you have to have good patience, you have to be very gentle, you have to be very quiet and you have to have good . . . good courage. } Ways of being that pacify
■ Gentle, quiet, patient

I: Good courage.

2. No information on validity and reliability was provided.

Activity 7—Evidence-Informed Practice Activity

The study response rate (52%) was relatively low but still acceptable. The findings are likely representative of the larger population and are therefore credible. However, when applying the study knowledge in making decisions, some caution will be needed, particularly as we examine the generalizability of the findings to nurses in other settings.

CHAPTER 15 QUALITATIVE DATA ANALYSIS

Activity 1
a. 3
b. 2
c. 5
d. 4
e. 1

Activity 2
Answers will vary.

Activity 3
Interpretation varies with every observer. The following is one interpretation of the text.

RP: Good courage. If you don't have good courage, sometimes things get in the way, but if you have good courage, everything is good for you.

I: That's an interesting word, courage.

RP: Yes, you have to have good courage. That is number one. Number two, you have to be very gentle, speak very quietly and have good courage. You know, when you have good courage you do everything for these people, like, this lady is my mother. I have to take good care of her.

Good Courage
- Ways of being that foster good outcomes
- Allows for genuine and authentic care that goes above and beyond

I: Okay.

RP: You know, so the work never feel hard. They never feel discouraged. You always have good energy to work.

I: Okay. Interesting. When I think of the word courage, I think of brave.

RP: Well, you call it, I say courage, good courage mean you have good energy, you have good strength, you're always happy to work.

I: Mm hmm.

Good Courage
- State of being that encompasses personal strength, happiness, positivity, harmony within the self
- Being present

RP: You have to have all these things in mind when you come to work. You focus on today is what I'm going to do for these people; so if you have the courage, you have the energy, your whole day is perfect.

I: And why is that so important on a special care unit?

RP: Because for me, I feel like I'm here to take good care of these people.

I: Mm hmm.

Context – connect ways of being to special care unit
- Purpose = care
- Caring can be challenging
- Good courage allow for the meeting of the challenge

RP: And I find myself feeling happy working with them. So when you're happy working with them, you know, you have a hard task, sometime it's very hard, sometime you have to have good courage, so you go and do everything every day to suit your needs.

I: What makes it hard on those days?

RP: Sometimes it's very hard, especially when you come like sundowning in the evenings.

I: Mm hmm.

RP: They're very restless, very aggressive. So you have to train yourself to know how to deal with these people. You can't talk to them hard, very quietly. Rub their shoulder, rub their back, and make them feel like they're at home.

Sundowning is a symptom of Alzheimer's disease. Confusion and agitation worsen in the late afternoon and evening, or as the sun goes down.

I: You train yourself.

RP: Yes, to do all these things to help them.

I: Can you tell me more about that? How do you train your-self?

RP: Well, okay. I'm coming to work today. This is what I want to do for this resident that I'm taking care of. If I came here and they are aggressive, I give them a drink of water; I'll give them a glass of juice if I can get a glass of juice. Then I put them to sit. I rub their hair a little bit, I rub their shoulder and so that way they don't feel left out.

I: Mm hmm.

Self Training
- Intention
- Thoughtful pacifying care
- Inclusion

Major Themes	Sub-Themes	Code
Good Courage	Pacifying ways of being	■ Gentle, quiet, patient
	■ Balancing ways of being	■ Ways of being that foster balance and energy ■ Ways of being that allows for genuine and authentic care ■ State of mind that fosters job satisfaction ■ State of being that encompasses personal strength, happiness, positivity, harmony within the self, and presence
	■ Presence	■ You have to have all these things in mind when you come to work. You focus on today is what I'm going to do for these people; so if you have the courage, you have the energy, your whole day is perfect.
	■ Living the everyday challenges	■ Managing the challenge of sundowning ■ Working with purpose ■ Working with intention ■ Inclusion

Activities 4 to 7
Answers will vary.

CHAPTER 16   QUANTITATIVE DATA ANALYSIS

Activity 1
You will have your set of completed cards.

Activity 2
1. a
2. c
3. d
4. a
5. a, b, or c, depending on the tool used to measure satisfaction
6. d

7. b
8. d
9. a
10. c

Activity 3

Across
1. j. Goofy's best friend
3. e. Old abbreviation for the mean
5. b. Abbreviation for the number of measures in a given data set (the measures may be individual people or some smaller pieces of data like blood pressure readings)
8. m. Describes a set of data with a standard deviation of 3 when compared with a set of data with a standard deviation of 12
10. h. Abbreviation for standard deviation
11. f. Marks the "score" where 50% of the scores are higher and 50% are lower
12. c. Measure of variation that shows the lowest and highest number in a dataset

Down
1. l. The values that occur most frequently in a data set
2. i. 68% of the values in a normal distribution fall between ±1 of this statistic
4. d. Can describe the height of a distribution
6. g. Describes a distribution characterized by a tail
7. k. Very unstable
9. a. Measure of central tendency used with interval of ratio data

Activity 4

1. a. IV = unknown
   b. DV = exercise participation, likely to be ratio/interval
2. a. IV = intervention, nominal
   b. DV = QOL, interval/ratio
   c. DV = cost, interval/ratio
3. a. IV = smoking status, nominal
   b. DV = depression, anxiety, stress, likely to be ratio/interval

Activity 5

1. Null hypothesis
2. ANOVA; parametric statistics
3. Measures of central tendency
4. Sampling error

5. Parameter; sample
6. Correlation
7. Type II error; type I error
8. Probability
9. Practical significance
10. Logistic regression analysis
11. Confidence interval
12. Research hypothesis; null hypothesis
13. c, b, a, e, d

Activity 6

1. Whether the childbirth experience or the preferred gender of the baby had an effect on the postpartum health scores
2. n, or the number of participants in each category, and the means and standard deviations of the scores on the postpartum health scale
3. t test
4. IV = childbirth experience, gender preferences; DV = postpartum health score
5. IV = nominal; DV = interval
6. There was no difference in postpartum health scores based on childbirth experience. There was no difference in postpartum health scores based on gender preference.

Activity 7

1. B. Yes
   C. Yes
2. B. Mean age, mean number of years as a registered nurse, number of males/females, highest level of education, unit specialty, employment status, and response rate.
   C. Nurses: roles (i.e., frontline nurses, managers, and educators), age range, nursing experience, level of education. Patients: age range, gender, ethnicity, employment status.
3. B. Yes, the descriptive statistics used were appropriate for the level of measurement.
   C. Yes, the descriptive information used was appropriate for this qualitative study
4. No
5. B. Yes
   C. No
6. B. A series of mediated multiple regression (ordinary least squares) analyses were conducted to examine the effects of bullying

and different sources of workplace incivility on patient outcomes through their effects on nurses' perception of patient safety risk.

C. N/A

7. The answers to this question may vary.

Activity 8—Web-Based Activity

1. Half of all women in Canada have experienced at least one incident of physical or sexual violence since the age of 16.
2. Within the context of spousal violence, three times as many women as men experience serious violence, such as choking, being beaten, being threatened with a knife or gun, and sexual violence. Furthermore, women are more likely to be physically injured, to get a restraining order, and to fear for their lives.

Activity 9—Evidence-Informed Practice Activity

Emergency department (ED) nurses should stop and consider how their actions in the ED could make a difference. They could check the websites listed as references on the Centers for Disease Control and Prevention (CDC) site and look for recommendations of experts in the field. They could anticipate finding guidelines for ways of interviewing injured women that would increase the probability of uncovering intimate partner violence (IPV). They could make sure that literature about IPV and safe places was readily available in the ED. They may also need to devise a way to keep some data so there could be some evaluation of the steps they had taken (such as by asking someone in the local school of nursing to work with them on this task).

CHAPTER 17   PRESENTING THE FINDINGS

Activity 1

1. R
2. D
3. R
4. D
5. R
6. R
7. R
8. D
9. D
10. D

Activity 2

1. Yes/No
   - The tables supplement the text.
   - They have precise headings and titles.
   - However, they repeat information already presented in the text.
2. A fact sheet by the Canadian Women's Foundation suggest that 50% of all women in Canada have experienced at least one incident of physical or sexual violence since the age of 16. Table 2 suggest that 39.1% and 66.3% of women in this sample have experienced nonphysical and physical violence, respectively. The study findings exceed the general population findings.
3. From the table provided, it appears that females were more likely to experience nonphysical violence.
4. From the table provided, it appears that males and females are equally as likely to experience childhood physical abuse.

Activity 3

Answers will vary from class to class.

Activity 4

1. a. Within the category "marital status," 137 of 247 women had never been married but were mothers. This is a total of 56.1% of the sample.
   b. The answer depends on the usual percentage of Native/Indigenous people that live in the area where the study was conducted. According to Statistics Canada, 309,845, or 22%, of the Indigenous identity population in Canada lived in Ontario in 2011. They make up 2.4% of the total population of that province. Since 2.4% of the general population of Ontarians could be categorized as Native/Indigenous and this study was conducted in Ontario, the number of Native/Indigenous people found in the study (5%) would be adequate.

c. Yes, Toronto is a diverse city, with about 50% of the current population being immigrants. So the sample would be representative of the general population.

2. a. Mean = 2.50. The score can range from 0 to 9. So across the group of 247 people, the average PTSD score was 2.50.

   b. ".710" tells us the strength and direction of the relationship between women's hyperarousal symptoms and avoidance/numbing symptoms. There is a strong relationship ($r > .6$ = a strong relationship) and a positive relationship (i.e., as hyperarousal scores increase, so do avoidance/numbing scores).

   c. 7

Activity 5—Web-Based Activity

1. The rating should be a 1; there were too many items to even think about reviewing, and there was very little consistency in the content among the items.

2. This answer will vary depending on when the search was conducted.

Activity 6—Evidence-Informed Practice Activity

Answers will vary depending on when the website was accessed and on personal experience.

CHAPTER 18   CRITIQUING QUALITATIVE RESEARCH

Activity 1

Appendix A: Answers will vary.
Appendix D: Answers will vary.

Activity 2

1. a. G
   b. B
   c. D
   d. A
   e. F
   f. D
   g. E
   h. G
   i. B

2. a. *Credibility* refers to qualitative research steps taken to ensure the accuracy, validity, and soundness of the data. Credibility can be confirmed when the research participants recognize the reported findings as their personal experience.

   b. *Auditability* is a research process that allows the work of a qualitative researcher or a person critiquing a research report to follow the thinking and/or conclusions of a researcher. The question of concern is whether the researcher(s) presented enough information for the reader to clearly understand the ways in which data were interpreted. When a data trail is auditable, it leads to the possibility of confirmability or the ability to clearly understand the ways in which the data were obtained, analyzed, and interpreted.

   c. *Fittingness* is the term used to answer these three questions: Are the findings applicable outside the study? Are the results or feelings meaningful to people not involved in the research? Are the findings meaningful to others who are in similar situations? Another idea closely related to fittingness is *transferability*: Can the findings be translated into similar experiences in meaningful ways?

   d. *Saturation* refers to the point at which data are being replicated such that no new ideas are coming forth about a specific concept or cultural phenomenon.

   e. *Trustworthiness* refers to the degree to which validity and reliability have been established; a research report is trustworthy when it accurately represents or portrays the participants' experience.

Activity 3—Web-Based Activity

Your instructor may want to direct you to view some specific Internet links to learn additional specific aspects of qualitative research.

Activity 4

1. narrative or quotes
2. trustworthiness
3. fittingness
4. emic
5. themes

CHAPTER 19 CRITIQUING QUANTITATIVE RESEARCH

Activity 1

Please note that what follows are the results of one inspectional reading of the article by Laschinger (2014). You are not expected to agree with these findings. Some of you may agree, but many of you will not.

Systematic skimming:
In reading the title, the abstract, the author affiliation, and the discussion, the following conclusions were made:

- The study fills a knowledge gap specifically related to the impact of workplace bullying on patient safety outcomes.
- The findings are interesting. This was the first study of its kind as per the authors and provides empirical support for the negative impact of workplace bullying and the ways in which it compromises patient safety. It is interesting that workplace bullying affects quality of care, which in turn impacts patient safety.
- A number of study limitations would significantly reduce the applicability of the finding. These include the design, which addresses relationships but not causation; the response rate, which will limit representativeness of the sample; and the fact that all nurses work in an acute care setting where there is much tension and pressure in the work environment. All of these factors limit the external validity of the findings.
- Caution would be needed in using the findings from this particular study, as the findings do not speak to cause and effect. Rather, they establish that when workplace bullying is perceived, patient care is compromised.

Answers to these questions will vary. Review possible responses with your instructor.

Superficial reading:
1. Fits my interest:
2. Remembered about the study:
3. Clinical or basic research:
4. Experimental, nonexperimental, or qualitative:
5. Rating on level-of-evidence scale:
6. Ethical questions:
Conclusion: I would reread this study in greater detail. It contains some nuggets that could support some interests of mine. It would not be directly related to my research interests, but it is interesting enough to be useful.

Remember, the purpose of inspectional reading is to decide what to do about further reading of the study. What did you decide?

CHAPTER 20 DEVELOPING AN EVIDENCE-INFORMED PRACTICE

Activity 1

Item #	Patient "P"	Intervention "I"	Comparison "C"	Outcome "O"	Time Frame "T"
#1	Parents	Recliners	Convert-O-Beds	More parents stay	Next 6 months
#2	Hemodialysis patients	Verbal instruction + take-home materials	Verbal instruction only	Decrease in adherence difficulties	Each visit
#3	Children	No vending machines	Vending machines	Decrease in weight of children	Past 5 years

Activity 2

Tool 1: PICOT

Tool 2: information literacy; librarian,

Tool 3: meta-analysis

Tool 4: therapy studies; meta-analysis; harm articles; confidence interval; relative-risk reduction; likelihood ratios

Tool 5: knowledge translation /dissemination

Activity 3—Web-Based Activity

1. In addition to gathering the best evidence, the systematic reviews will also contain evidence that is still easy to obtain and may not be published.

2. Searches take place online and can be completed by using keywords, topics, review groups, authors, and date-range.

3. Through subscription (individual or institutional) to the Cochrane Library at www. thecochranelibrary.com, CD-ROM, or by pay-per-view

4. Answers will vary.

5. Answers will vary.

NOTES

NOTES